T0245216

Hyperparathyroidism

Ann E. Kearns
Robert A. Wermers
Editors

Hyperparathyroidism

A Clinical Casebook

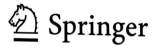 Springer

Editors
Ann E. Kearns
Mayo Clinic
Rochester, MN, USA

Robert A. Wermers
Mayo Clinic
Rochester, MN, USA

ISBN 978-3-319-25878-2   ISBN 978-3-319-25880-5   (eBook)
DOI 10.1007/978-3-319-25880-5

Library of Congress Control Number: 2016930302

Springer Cham Heidelberg New York Dordrecht London
© Mayo Foundation for Medical Education and Research 2016
This work is subject to copyright. All rights are reserved by the Publisher, whether
the whole or part of the material is concerned, specifically the rights of translation,
reprinting, reuse of illustrations, recitation, broadcasting, reproduction on microfilms
or in any other physical way, and transmission or information storage and retrieval,
electronic adaptation, computer software, or by similar or dissimilar methodology
now known or hereafter developed.
The use of general descriptive names, registered names, trademarks, service marks,
etc. in this publication does not imply, even in the absence of a specific statement, that
such names are exempt from the relevant protective laws and regulations and therefore free for general use.
The publisher, the authors and the editors are safe to assume that the advice and
information in this book are believed to be true and accurate at the date of publication. Neither the publisher nor the authors or the editors give a warranty, express or
implied, with respect to the material contained herein or for any errors or omissions
that may have been made.

Printed on acid-free paper

Springer International Publishing AG Switzerland is part of Springer
Science+Business Media (www.springer.com)

Preface

Once you start studying medicine, you never get through with it.
Charles H. Mayo, MD

The practice of medicine is one of continuous learning through clinical experience. In this volume, we have collected observations obtained through the clinical practice of expert clinicians. Each chapter begins with a case history, which describes insights into the disease of hyperparathyroidism, use of diagnostic tests in its evaluation, implementation of medical and surgical therapeutic interventions, and clinical outcomes. This approach is a useful real-life approach to learning through the patient encounters physicians have every day.

The contributing authors were encouraged to choose cases that provide relevant pearls and highlight the state of the art of patient management. Reasoned opinion is provided when evidence is less clear. The hope is that this format stimulates the self-directed learning, centered on patient care questions, that is the hallmark of the profession of medicine and that is relevant to learners at all levels of experience.

We would like to acknowledge the authors for their work in putting together their collective experiences and observations to share with others. We also want to thank the patients who provided and continue to provide the inspiration to ask questions and seek answers, to ultimately continue learning.

Rochester, MN, USA   Ann E. Kearns, MD, PhD
                                       Robert A. Wermers, MD

Contents

Contributors

EeeLN H. Buckarma, MD Department of Surgery, Mayo College of Medicine, Mayo Clinic, Rochester, MN, USA

Bart L. Clarke, MD Division of Endocrinology, Diabetes, Metabolism, and Nutrition, Department of Internal Medicine, Mayo College of Medicine, Mayo Clinic, Rochester, MN, USA

Danae A. Delivanis, MD Division of Endocrinology, Diabetes, Metabolism, and Nutrition, Department of Internal Medicine, Mayo College of Medicine, Mayo Clinic, Rochester, MN, USA

Matthew T. Drake, MD, PhD Division of Endocrinology, Diabetes, Metabolism, and Nutrition, Department of Internal Medicine, Mayo College of Medicine, Mayo Clinic, Rochester, MN, USA

Lori A. Erickson, MD Department of Laboratory Medicine and Pathology, Mayo College of Medicine, Mayo Clinic, Rochester, MN, USA

David R. Farley, MD Department of Surgery, Mayo College of Medicine, Mayo Clinic, Rochester, MN, USA

Stefan K. Grebe, MD, PhD Department of Laboratory Medicine and Pathology, Mayo College of Medicine, Mayo Clinic, Rochester, MN, USA

Marcio L. Griebeler, MD Department of Internal Medicine, Sanford University of South Dakota Medical Center, Sioux Falls, SD, USA

Daniel L. Hurley, MD Division of Endocrinology, Diabetes, Metabolism, and Nutrition, Department of Internal Medicine, Mayo College of Medicine, Mayo Clinic, Rochester, MN, USA

Johann P. Ingimarsson, MD Department of Urology, Mayo College of Medicine, Mayo Clinic, Rochester, MN, USA

Nicole M. Iñiguez-Ariza, MD Division of Endocrinology, Diabetes, Metabolism, and Nutrition, Department of Internal Medicine, Mayo College of Medicine, Mayo Clinic, Rochester, MN, USA

Haleigh James, MD Division of Endocrinology, Diabetes, Metabolism, and Nutrition, Department of Internal Medicine, Mayo College of Medicine, Mayo Clinic, Rochester, MN, USA

Ann E. Kearns, MD, PhD Division of Endocrinology, Diabetes, Metabolism, and Nutrition, Department of Internal Medicine, Mayo College of Medicine, Mayo Clinic, Rochester, MN, USA

Kurt A. Kennel, MD Division of Endocrinology, Diabetes, Metabolism, and Nutrition, Department of Internal Medicine, Mayo College of Medicine, Mayo Clinic, Rochester, MN, USA

John C. Lieske, MD Division of Nephrology and Hypertension, Department of Internal Medicine, Mayo College of Medicine, Mayo Clinic, Rochester, MN, USA

Hana Barbra Lo, MD Division of Endocrinology, Department of Pediatric and Adolescent Medicine, Mayo Clinic, Rochester, MN, USA

Travis J. McKenzie, MD Department of Surgery, Mayo College of Medicine, Mayo Clinic, Rochester, MN, USA

Manpreet S. Mundi, MD Division of Endocrinology, Diabetes, Metabolism, and Nutrition, Department of Internal Medicine, Mayo College of Medicine, Mayo Clinic, Rochester, MN, USA

Naykky Singh Ospina, MD Division of Endocrinology, Diabetes, Metabolism, and Nutrition, Department of Internal Medicine, Mayo College of Medicine, Mayo Clinic, Rochester, MN, USA

T. K. Pandian, MD, MPH Division of Subspecialty General Surgery, Department of Surgery, Mayo College of Medicine, Mayo Clinic, Rochester, MN, USA

Melanie L. Richards, MD, MHPE Department of Surgery, Mayo College of Medicine, Mayo Clinic, Rochester, MN, USA

Jad G. Sfeir, MD Division of Endocrinology, Diabetes, Metabolism, and Nutrition, Department of Internal Medicine, Mayo College of Medicine, Mayo Clinic, Rochester, MN, USA

Omair A. Shariq, MRCS Department of Surgery, Mayo Clinic, Rochester, MN, USA

Peter J. Tebben, MD Division of Endocrinology, Department of Pediatric and Adolescent Medicine, Mayo Clinic, Rochester, MN, USA

Division of Endocrinology, Diabetes, Metabolism, and Nutrition, Department of Internal Medicine, Mayo College of Medicine, Mayo Clinic, Rochester, MN, USA

Geoffrey B. Thompson, MD Department of Surgery, Mayo College of Medicine, Mayo Clinic, Rochester, MN, USA

Nishanth Vallumsetla, MBBS Division of Endocrinology, Diabetes, Metabolism, and Nutrition, Department of Internal Medicine, Mayo College of Medicine, Mayo Clinic, Rochester, MN, USA

Robert A. Wermers, MD Division of Endocrinology, Diabetes, Metabolism, and Nutrition, Department of Internal Medicine, Mayo College of Medicine, Mayo Clinic, Rochester, MN, USA

Chapter 1
Asymptomatic Primary Hyperparathyroidism

Danae A. Delivanis and Robert A. Wermers

Case Presentation

A 65-year-old female was referred for evaluation of primary hyperparathyroidism (PHPT). Review of symptoms was significant for a 7-month history of bilateral shoulder pain as well as bilateral lower extremity muscle aches. An evaluation by rheumatology, including a workup for inflammatory processes, was unrevealing. A 6-week trial of corticosteroids for possible polymyalgia rheumatica was given with some improvement of symptomatology. The patient denied polyuria, polydipsia, abdominal pain, fatigue, or constipation. Her mood was stable.

A laboratory investigation revealed hypercalcemia with a serum calcium – 10.3 mg/dL (nl, 8.9–10.1), phosphorus – 4.2 mg/dL (nl, 2.5–4.5), creatinine – 1.0 mg/dL with an estimated GFR >60 mL/min/BSA, intact parathyroid hormone (PTH) – 68 pg/mL (nl 15–65), and 25-hydroxyvitamin D – 28 ng/mL. Upon

D.A. Delivanis, MD • R.A. Wermers, MD (✉)
Division of Endocrinology, Diabetes, Metabolism, and Nutrition,
Department of Internal Medicine, Mayo College of Medicine,
Mayo Clinic, Rochester, MN, USA
e-mail: Delivanis.danae@mayo.edu; wermers.robert@mayo.edu

A.E. Kearns, R.A. Wermers (eds.), *Hyperparathyroidism:*
A Clinical Casebook, DOI 10.1007/978-3-319-25880-5_1,
© Mayo Foundation for Medical Education and Research 2016

further review of her electronic medical record, calcium levels have been persistently elevated over the last 5 months with a maximum calcium elevation of 10.4 mg/dL.

She was not on hydrochlorothiazide or lithium and did not have a history of prior lithium use, but was on a transdermal estrogen patch 0.05 mg/24 h weekly, which was often not removed for 3–4 weeks at a time. She denied a history of head or neck radiation. Her daily dietary calcium intake was estimated at 600 mg in addition to a daily multivitamin, and she denied both calcium and vitamin D supplementation. Her family history was negative for hypercalcemia or familial parathyroid syndromes.

Her past medical history was negative for fragility fractures, but she did believe she had some height loss. She denied a history of nephrolithiasis. A dual-energy X-ray absorptiometry (DXA) bone mineral density (BMD) was done 3 years prior and revealed well-preserved bone at the spine and hip by patient report.

Assessment and Diagnosis

The most common presentation of PHPT is asymptomatic hypercalcemia. Indeed, in the most recent population-based study on the epidemiology of PHPT, from 1998 to 2010 only 11 % of community-dwelling patients presented with symptoms [1]. The diagnosis is usually first suspected through the incidental finding of an elevated serum calcium concentration on biochemical screening tests. More recently, an increased incidence of PHPT has been observed, likely due to case ascertainment bias from targeted screening in patients being evaluated for osteoporosis [1]. PHPT is usually confirmed with a concomitant elevation in calcium and PTH concentration or when PTH is in the normal range but inappropriately when associated with hypercalcemia. It is important to understand that the diagnosis of PHPT is made through biochemical evaluation. Localization studies should only be considered when the decision to proceed with a surgical approach has been made.

Factors complicating the biochemical diagnosis of PHPT include fluctuation of serum calcium and PTH levels that can be seen in patients. It is well recognized that in normal individuals, PTH secretion is dynamic in nature, with intermittent pulses superimposed upon a background basal secretion [2]. Also, PTH secretion has a circadian rhythm [3], and nonsteady-state perturbations of the parathyroid glands have dramatic effects on PTH secretion [4]. In subjects with PHPT, PTH secretion and expression can be modified by several external factors [5, 6]. In addition, a significant inverse relationship between parathyroid gland weight and 25-hydroxyvitamin D levels exists, revealing that vitamin D deficiency can be associated with more severe disease [7]. Finally, vitamin D repletion in patients with PHPT can decrease levels of PTH and bone turnover [8].

Before PHPT is diagnosed, patients may exhibit evidence of mild abnormalities in calcium homeostasis. As an example, a population-based study performing screening serum calcium measurements in 5771 postmenopausal women from Sweden identified 230 women (4.4 %) with high normal serum calcium results or hypercalcemia without clear criteria for PHPT. Subsequent evaluation more than 8 years later observed that 45 % of these women met diagnostic criteria for PHPT [9]. Normocalcemic PHPT is defined by a normal serum calcium and elevated PTH without a secondary cause of the PHPT such as hypovitaminosis D, chronic kidney disease (CKD), or hyper-calciuria (see Chap. 18) [10]. Patients with normocalcemic PHPT have similar clinical characteristics to PHPT including that most with this disorder are postmenopausal women. In addition, a significant number of patients with normocalcemic PHPT subsequently develop hypercalcemia (19 %) [10] and clinical complications similar to those seen in hypercalcemic PHPT [11, 12].

Management

Although patients with symptomatic PHPT should consider parathyroid surgery, the widespread identification of asymptomatic individuals raises the question of need for and timing of surgical intervention in this population. Based on the most recent guidelines [13], several tests are recommended to assess the most appropriate clinical management. Measurement of serum creatinine and estimated glomerular filtration rate (eGFR) as well as imaging studies of the kidneys to screen for occult kidney stones are recommended evaluations for potential renal complications related to PHPT. In order to distinguish PHPT from familial benign hypocalciuric hypercalcemia (FHH) and also to determine risk of kidney stones, a measurement of a 24-h urinary calcium and creatinine should be considered. In addition, to assess for osteoporosis possibly related to PHPT, DXA BMD of the spine, hip, and wrist and imaging to screen for presence of vertebral compression fractures is suggested. Finally, measurement of 25-hydroxyvitamin D is useful since vitamin D deficiency is highly prevalent in PHPT and if present can increase the PTH measurement [14].

The indications for parathyroid surgery, in an otherwise asymptomatic PHPT patient, are shown in Table 1.1 as presented in the Fourth International Workshop on this condition [13]. Fulfilling one of the criteria is sufficient to recommend a surgical approach. These guidelines have been proposed to help the provider and patient decide on the advisability of parathyroid surgery. However, there are several cases where clinical judgment should be applied. For example, in an elderly patient with asymptomatic PHPT and a slight age-related decrease in GFR, observation may be appropriate. In the same way, older individuals with increased fracture risk and mild hypercalcemia without fragility fractures may consider osteoporosis medical therapy rather than parathyroidectomy.

Table 1.1 Guidelines for surgery in asymptomatic primary hyperparathyroidism

Assessment	
Serum calcium (> upper limit of normal)	1.0 mg/dL (0.25 mmol/L)
Skeletal	Bone mineral density: T-score ≤2.5 at lumbar spine, total hip, femoral neck, or distal 1/3 radius
	Vertebral fracture by imaging
Renal	Creatinine clearance <60 mL/min
	24-h urine calcium >400 mg/day (>10 mmol/day) and increased stone risk by biochemical stone risk analysis
	Presence of nephrolithiasis or nephrocalcinosis by radiograph, ultrasound, or computed tomography
Age (years)	<50

Adapted from the Fourth International Workshop of asymptomatic primary hyperparathyroidism [13]

Regarding calcium and vitamin D intake for patients with asymptomatic PHPT, studies have shown that there is no indication for dietary calcium restriction; 800–1000 mg daily dietary calcium intake is recommended, but less may be considered in patients with hypercalciuria [15]. In addition, vitamin D-deficient patients with PHPT have been shown to have higher levels of PTH, markers of bone turnover, and more frequent fractures than vitamin D-replete patients [14]. Vitamin D repletion in patients with PHPT doesn't exacerbate hypercalcemia and low serum 25-hydroxyvitamin D should be replaced with vitamin D supplementation aiming to bring the serum 25-hydroxyvitamin D levels to the level of at least 20 ng/mL [8, 16].

In this case, a DXA BMD revealed osteopenia at the total hip and femur neck with T-scores of −1.1 and −1.5, respectively, well-preserved bone density at the lumbar spine with a T-score of −0.1, and a nondominant left one-third radius T-score of −0.9.

Spine radiographs did not reveal compressive fractures. Her 10-year risks for a major osteoporotic fracture and hip fracture were 10 % and 1.5 %, respectively. Imaging of her kidneys was negative for urinary calculi. Her 25-hydroxyvitamin D deficiency level was sufficient. A 24-h urine calcium was 135 mg with a fractional excretion of filtered calcium of 0.014, which in conjunction with a negative family history of hypercalcemia made FHH unlikely.

After completion of the initial evaluation, the patient was seen for follow-up to determine management of her mild and uncomplicated PHPT. The natural history of mild PHPT suggests that progression can occur, such that by 15 years of prospective follow-up, as many as one-third of subjects will demonstrate more overt features of the disease (e.g., kidney stones, worsening hypercalcemia, and reduced BMD) [17]. Hence, surgery should be considered in patients for whom medical surveillance is not desired. In addition, compared to observation, successful parathyroid surgery is associated with spine and hip bone density improvement [18], reduced rate of nephrolithiasis among those with a history of renal stone disease [19], and there may be improvement in some neurocognitive elements [20–22]. In these cases, an informed discussion needs to be had and patient's preference is pivotal for a shared decision-making approach. With advances in the effectiveness and safety of surgical techniques, particularly in the hands of expert parathyroid surgeons [23, 24], the decision to remove the abnormal parathyroid tissue is often reinforced by the added confidence of its success and limited risk of postoperative complications.

Given the patient's ongoing symptoms of lower extremity pain as well as concern of long-term complications and progression of PHPT, she elected to consider parathyroid surgery and meet with an experienced endocrine surgeon. A parathyroid scan was subsequently performed, but was non-localizing. After her appointment with the surgeon, she elected to observe, rather

Table 1.2 Guidelines for monitoring observed patients with mild asymptomatic primary hyperparathyroidism

Assessment	
Serum calcium	Annually
Skeletal	Bone mineral density every 1–2 years (spine, hip, wrist)
	Imaging of spine if clinically indicated (e.g., height loss, back pain)
Renal	eGFR, serum creatinine annually
	If renal stones suspected, 24-h biochemical stone profile, renal imaging by X-ray, ultrasound, or computed tomography

Adapted in part from the Fourth International Workshop of asymptomatic primary hyperparathyroidism [13]

to proceed with parathyroidectomy. Asymptomatic patients who do not undergo surgery require monitoring for worsening hypercalcemia, renal impairment, and bone loss. The development of any of these findings may indicate disease progression and the reconsideration of surgical intervention. The Fourth International Workshop [13] recommendations for monitoring asymptomatic PHPT are outlined in Table 1.2.

Outcome

Repeat laboratory investigations and a follow-up visit were scheduled in a year time interval. Given the fact that level of 25-hydroxyvitamin D was 28 ng/mL, it was recommended to continue with dietary intake of vitamin D 800 IU daily and as well maintain a moderate dietary calcium intake of about 1000 mg/day. Finally, the patient was instructed to avoid dehydration and to contact us if any problems related to PHPT occurred in the interim.

Clinical Pearls/Pitfalls
- Most PHPT patients in the community are asymptomatic and identified incidentally through a serum calcium measurement.
- An evaluation of PHPT-related complications should be performed prior to deciding upon management.
- Patients who do not meet surgical criteria or are unable or unwilling to proceed with parathyroidectomy should be monitored on an annual basis, since over time approximately one-third of patients will demonstrate disease progression.
- Parathyroid localization is not used to diagnose PHPT and should only be ordered if surgery is decided upon through a shared decision-making approach.
- Consider the possibility of FHH before referring the patient for possible parathyroid surgery.

Conflicts of Interest All authors state that they have no conflicts of interest.

References

1. Griebeler ML, Kearns AE, Ryu E, Hathcock MA, Melton 3rd LJ, Wermers RA. Secular trends in the incidence of primary hyperparathyroidism over five decades (1965–2010). Bone. 2015;73:1–7.
2. Samuels MH, Veldhuis J, Cawley C, Urban RJ, Luther M, Bauer R, et al. Pulsatile secretion of parathyroid hormone in normal young subjects: assessment by deconvolution analysis. J Clin Endocrinol Metab. 1993;77(2):399–403.
3. Calvo MS, Eastell R, Offord KP, Bergstralh EJ, Burritt MF. Circadian variation in ionized calcium and intact parathyroid hormone: evidence for sex differences in calcium homeostasis. J Clin Endocrinol Metab. 1991;72(1):69–76.

4. Schmitt CP, Schaefer F, Bruch A, Veldhuis JD, Schmidt-Gayk H, Stein G, et al. Control of pulsatile and tonic parathyroid hormone secretion by ionized calcium. J Clin Endocrinol Metab. 1996;81(12):4236–43.
5. Insogna KL, Mitnick ME, Stewart AF, Burtis WJ, Mallette LE, Broadus AE. Sensitivity of the parathyroid hormone-1,25-dihydroxyvitamin D axis to variations in calcium intake in patients with primary hyperparathyroidism. N Engl J Med. 1985;313(18):1126–30.
6. Tohme JF, Bilezikian JP, Clemens TL, Silverberg SJ, Shane E, Lindsay R. Suppression of parathyroid hormone secretion with oral calcium in normal subjects and patients with primary hyperparathyroidism. J Clin Endocrinol Metab. 1990;70(4):951–6.
7. Rao DS, Honasoge M, Divine GW, Phillips ER, Lee MW, Ansari MR, et al. Effect of vitamin D nutrition on parathyroid adenoma weight: pathogenetic and clinical implications. J Clin Endocrinol Metab. 2000;85(3):1054–8.
8. Grey A, Lucas J, Horne A, Gamble G, Davidson JS, Reid IR. Vitamin D repletion in patients with primary hyperparathyroidism and coexistent vitamin D insufficiency. J Clin Endocrinol Metab. 2005;90(4):2122–6.
9. Lundgren E, Hagstrom EG, Lundin J, Winnerback K, Roos J, Ljunghall S, et al. Primary hyperparathyroidism revisited in menopausal women with serum calcium in the upper normal range at population-based screening 8 years ago. World J Surg. 2002;26(8):931–6.
10. Lowe H, McMahon DJ, Rubin MR, Bilezikian JP, Silverberg SJ. Normocalcemic primary hyperparathyroidism: further characterization of a new clinical phenotype. J Clin Endocrinol Metab. 2007;92(8):3001–5.
11. Tuna MM, Caliskan M, Unal M, Demirci T, Dogan BA, Kucukler K, et al. Normocalcemic hyperparathyroidism is associated with complications similar to those of hypercalcemic hyperparathyroidism. J Bone Miner Metab. 2015 [ahead of print].
12. Chen G, Xue Y, Zhang Q, Xue T, Yao J, Huang H, et al. Is normocalcemic primary hyperparathyroidism harmful or harmless? J Clin Endocrinol Metab. 2015;100(6):2420–4.
13. Bilezikian JP, Brandi ML, Eastell R, Silverberg SJ, Udelsman R, Marcocci C, et al. Guidelines for the management of asymptomatic primary hyperparathyroidism: summary statement from the Fourth International Workshop. J Clin Endocrinol Metab. 2014;99(10):3561–9.
14. Silverberg SJ, Shane E, Dempster DW, Bilezikian JP. The effects of vitamin D insufficiency in patients with primary hyperparathyroidism. Am J Med. 1999;107(6):561–7.

15. Locker FG, Silverberg SJ, Bilezikian JP. Optimal dietary calcium intake in primary hyperparathyroidism. J Clin Endocrinol Metab. 1997;102(6):543–50.
16. Marcocci C, Bollerslev J, Khan AA, Shoback DM. Medical management of primary hyperparathyroidism: proceedings of the fourth International Workshop on the Management of Asymptomatic Primary Hyperparathyroidism. J Clin Endocrinol Metab. 2014;99(10):3607–18.
17. Rubin MR, Bilezikian JP, McMahon DJ, Jacobs T, Shane E, Siris E, et al. The natural history of primary hyperparathyroidism with or without parathyroid surgery after 15 years. J Clin Endocrinol Metab. 2008;93(9):3462–70.
18. Silverberg SJ, Shane E, Jacobs TP, Siris E, Bilezikian JP. A 10-year prospective study of primary hyperparathyroidism with or without parathyroid surgery. N Engl J Med. 1999;341(17):1249–55.
19. Mollerup CL, Vestergaard P, Frokjaer VG, Mosekilde L, Christiansen P, Blichert-Toft M. Risk of renal stone events in primary hyperparathyroidism before and after parathyroid surgery: controlled retrospective follow up study. BMJ. 2002;325(7368):807.
20. Zanocco K, Butt Z, Kaltman D, Elaraj D, Cella D, Holl JL, et al. Improvement in patient-reported physical and mental health after parathyroidectomy for primary hyperparathyroidism. Surgery. 2015;158: 837–45.
21. Espiritu RP, Kearns AE, Vickers KS, Grant C, Ryu E, Wermers RA. Depression in primary hyperparathyroidism: prevalence and benefit of surgery. J Clin Endocrinol Metab. 2011;96(11):E1737–45.
22. Weber T, Eberle J, Messelhauser U, Schiffmann L, Nies C, Schabram J, et al. Parathyroidectomy, elevated depression scores, and suicidal ideation in patients with primary hyperparathyroidism: results of a prospective multicenter study. JAMA Surg. 2013;148(2):109–15.
23. Stavrakis AI, Ituarte PH, Ko CY, Yeh MW. Surgeon volume as a predictor of outcomes in inpatient and outpatient endocrine surgery. Surgery. 2007;142(6):887–99; discussion -99.
24. Mitchell J, Milas M, Barbosa G, Sutton J, Berber E, Siperstein A. Avoidable reoperations for thyroid and parathyroid surgery: effect of hospital volume. Surgery. 2008;144(6):899–906; discussion -7.

Chapter 2
Severe Primary Hyperparathyroidism

Ann E. Kearns

Case Presentation

A 58-year-old female with a history of Hodgkin lymphoma treated with chemotherapy 20 years prior presented with left leg pain after a fall from standing height. Physical exam was notable for deformity of the left lower extremity and a large left-sided neck mass. Left hip x-ray confirmed a subtrochanteric femur fracture and a lytic lesion. Lucent lesions were noted on the left femoral shaft and patella (Fig. 2.1). Computed tomography (CT) scan of the chest, abdomen, and pelvis was notable for a 3.5×2.5 cm peritracheal nodule with local compression of the trachea. Widespread "metastatic" lytic lesions were noted diffusely throughout the axial and appendicular skeleton, and non-obstructing calyceal tip stones were also present. Laboratory results revealed a serum calcium of 15.6 mg/dL (8.9–10.2 mg/dL), alkaline phosphatase of 399 units/L (46–118 U/L), and a mild normocytic anemia.

A.E. Kearns, MD, PhD
Division of Endocrinology, Diabetes, Metabolism, and Nutrition,
Department of Internal Medicine, Mayo College of Medicine,
Mayo Clinic, Rochester, MN, USA
e-mail: kearns.ann@mayo.edu

A.E. Kearns, R.A. Wermers (eds.), *Hyperparathyroidism:*
A Clinical Casebook, DOI 10.1007/978-3-319-25880-5_2,
© Mayo Foundation for Medical Education and Research 2016

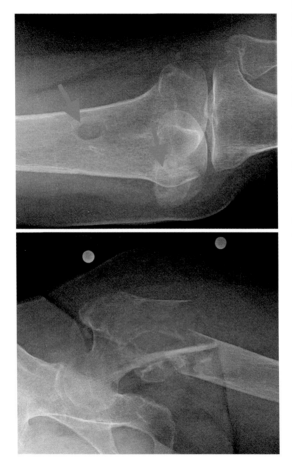

Fig. 2.1 (*Left*) X-ray of left femur showing subtrochanteric fracture and lytic lesion. (*Right*) X-ray of left distal femur showing lucent lesions (*arrows*)

Her hypercalcemia was treated with aggressive intravenous fluid administration, subcutaneous calcitonin, and zoledronic acid 4 mg. Her calcium level normalized. An ultrasound of the neck showed a solid mass encompassing the left lobe of the thyroid with sonographic features of malignancy. Parathyroid hormone (PTH) was 1510 pg/mL (15–65 pg/mL), and 25-hydroxyvitamin D was undetectable. The thyroid-stimulating hormone (TSH) level was 3.5 mIU/L (0.3–5.0 mIU/L). Fine-needle aspiration (FNA) of the neck mass was positive for neoplastic cells with Hürthle cell features.

Assessment and Diagnosis

The most likely diagnosis for a patient presenting with a pathologic fracture, lytic bone lesions, and severe hypercalcemia is widespread malignancy. The presence of a neck mass would also be consistent with a malignancy. The cytology of FNA does not prove or disprove malignancy. Although thyroid cancers such as follicular, medullary, or anaplastic thyroid carcinoma can metastasize to the bone, they are not generally associated with hypercalcemia. The profound elevation of PTH indicates a PTH-mediated hypercalcemia. The findings of severe hypercalcemia, significant elevation of PTH, and a neck mass are highly suspicious for parathyroid carcinoma [1–3]. Cytologic features alone on FNA cannot distinguish thyroid and parathyroid tissue nor parathyroid carcinoma from benign parathyroid tissue.

Lytic bone lesions are a common finding when widespread malignancy metastasizes to the bone and also in multiple myeloma which can also result in severe hypercalcemia. Osteitis fibrosa cystica is a skeletal disorder with lytic bone lesions related to hyperparathyroidism. Although rarely seen in the USA today, it occurs in severe long-standing primary hyperparathyroidism and parathyroid carcinoma. The proliferation and activity of osteoclasts in response to PTH leads to cystic defects that can produce pain and be locally aggressive, resulting in pathologic fractures. This is often initially mistaken for widespread malignancy [4]. However, the lesions are composed of numerous multinucleated giant cells admixed with fibroblasts and associated with interstitial hemorrhage marked by hemosiderin deposition, resulting in a brown appearance ("brown tumors"). The imaging and histology in isolation may not be diagnostic for osteitis fibrosa cystica due to overlapping features with other conditions but in addition to the biochemical and clinical picture, can lead to the correct diagnosis.

When parathyroid carcinoma is a concern, as in this setting, the surgical team should be alerted to this possibility so that the appropriate en bloc surgical resection can be performed (see Chap. 10). Also when parathyroid carcinoma is a concern, FNA is not diagnostic and has the potential for tumor seeding [5].

Management

The subtrochanteric femur fracture required resection and endoprosthetic replacement. The pathology from the operation revealed a brown tumor of hyperparathyroidism (Fig. 2.2). The patient then underwent neck surgery with excision of a 5.3×3.5×2.2 cm left superior parathyroid adenoma that was adherent to the left lobe of the thyroid but did not show invasion to suggest carcinoma. Postoperatively, hypocalcemia and hypophosphatemia developed, and she was treated with calcium, initially intravenous via central line, and calcitriol.

Hypocalcemia following parathyroidectomy is common but usually transient and not symptomatic. Hungry bone syndrome is the term used to describe prolonged, severe, symptomatic hypocalcemia, often with hypophosphatemia, accompanied by

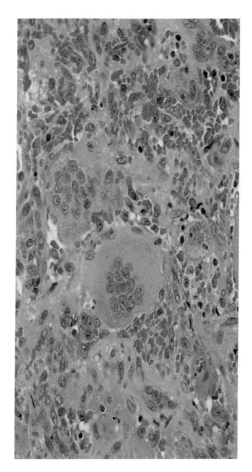

Fig. 2.2 Histology of tumor-resected femur showing the presence of multinucleated giant cells admixed with fibroblasts and associated with interstitial hemorrhage consistent with a brown tumor from hyperparathyroidism

normal or elevated PTH levels [6]. This distinguishes it from postoperative hypoparathyroidism in which the PTH is low and the phosphorus is increased. Depending on the severity of hypercalcemia at the time of surgery, the development of hypocalcemia due to hypoparathyroidism may be delayed up to 48 h postoperatively. Postoperative hypoparathyroidism is often also accompanied by significant hypercalciuria, due to the loss of PTH-stimulated renal tubular reabsorption of calcium, and is not seen in hungry bone syndrome. The hypophosphatemia of hungry bone syndrome does not usually require replacement (unless <1.0 mg/dL), and intravenous phosphorus should be avoided due to the further lowering of calcium seen with it. In this case, hypocalcemia developed rapidly following parathyroidectomy, as her calcium was normalized preoperatively. Her coexistent vitamin D deficiency may also have contributed to hungry bone syndrome.

Reduction in bone resorption and increase in bone formation occur acutely after removal of the abnormal parathyroid tissue, resulting in the large influx of calcium into the bone. Although the incidence of hungry bone syndrome is not well defined, an older case series identified the volume of resected parathyroid adenoma, preoperative blood urea nitrogen, preoperative alkaline phosphatase, and older age as predictors of its development [7]. The presence of bone disease also is a risk factor [6]. The treatment of hungry bone syndrome requires calcium (sometimes intravenous) and calcitriol and may last for months. The use of bisphosphonates to lower bone remodeling and prevent the development of hungry bone syndrome has been reported in small series [8–10]. Our patient did receive preoperative zoledronic acid but still developed hungry bone syndrome. In contrast to bisphosphonates, preoperative cinacalcet therapy in secondary hyperparathyroidism may be a risk for lower calcium postoperatively [11, 12]. Prospective trials have not been performed to inform the optimal treatment or prevention of hungry bone syndrome.

Outcome

Over the 6 months following dismissal from the hospital, hypocalcemia resolved and calcitriol was discontinued. The bone lesions showed sclerosis consistent with interval healing.

> **Clinical Pearls/Pitfalls**
> - Severe bone disease from PHPT (osteitis fibrosa cystica) can mimic metastatic malignancy.
> - Cytology on FNA cannot distinguish thyroid tissue from parathyroid tissue nor benign parathyroid tissue from parathyroid carcinoma.
> - A prior FNA can make histologic assessment of invasion difficult due to biopsy site changes and has a remote risk for tumor rupture or seeding tumor cells.
> - Postoperative hypocalcemia from hungry bone syndrome is more likely in patients with severe long-standing hyperparathyroidism and evidence of related bone disease.

Conflict of Interest All authors state that they have no conflicts of interest.

References

1. Shane E. Clinical review 122: parathyroid carcinoma. J Clin Endocrinol Metab. 2001;86(2):485–93.
2. Wynne AG, et al. Parathyroid carcinoma: clinical and pathologic features in 43 patients. Medicine. 1992;71(4):197–205.
3. Robert JH, et al. Primary hyperparathyroidism: can parathyroid carcinoma be anticipated on clinical and biochemical grounds? Report of

nine cases and review of the literature. Ann Surg Oncol. 2005;12(7): 526–32.

4. Yang Q, et al. Skeletal lesions in primary hyperparathyroidism. Am J Med Sci. 2015;349(4):321–7.

5. Spinelli C, et al. Cutaneous spreading of parathyroid carcinoma after fine needle aspiration cytology. J Endocrinol Invest. 2000;23(4): 255–7.

6. Witteveen JE, et al. Hungry bone syndrome: still a challenge in the post-operative management of primary hyperparathyroidism: a systematic review of the literature. Eur J Endocrinol/Eur Fed Endocr Soc. 2013;168(3):R45–53.

7. Brasier AR, Nussbaum SR. Hungry bone syndrome: clinical and biochemical predictors of its occurrence after parathyroid surgery. Am J Med. 1988;84(4):654–60.

8. Lee IT, et al. Bisphosphonate pretreatment attenuates hungry bone syndrome postoperatively in subjects with primary hyperparathyroidism. J Bone Miner Metab. 2006;24(3):255–8.

9. Kumar A, Ralston SH. Bisphosphonates prevent the hungry bone syndrome. Nephron. 1996;74(4):729.

10. Davenport A, Stearns MP. Administration of pamidronate helps prevent immediate postparathyroidectomy hungry bone syndrome. Nephrology. 2007;12(4):386–90.

11. Wirowski D, et al. Cinacalcet effects on the perioperative course of patients with secondary hyperparathyroidism. Langenbeck's Arch Surg/Deut Ges Chir. 2013;398(1):131–8.

12. Meyers MO, et al. Postoperative hypocalcemia after parathyroidectomy for renal hyperparathyroidism in the era of cinacalcet. Am Surg. 2009;75(9):843–7.

Chapter 3
Nephrolithiasis in Primary Hyperparathyroidism

Johann P. Ingimarsson and John C. Lieske

Case Presentation

A 73-year-old female is incidentally found to have five right and two left 1–5 mm calyceal kidney stones on an abdominal ultrasound that are confirmed on a subsequent CT scan, both performed for an abdominal pain thought to be biliary in origin. She has no known history of passing kidney stones, but did have an episode of severe crampy abdominal and flank pain some years prior which resolved. Her past medical history is significant for cervical cancer at age 35, hysterectomy, bilateral knee replacement, gastritis, bronchitis, and insomnia. Her two children both have had symptomatic kidney stones. She is not on any lithogenic medications or thiazide diuretics. She is found to have serum calcium of 10.6 mg/dL (nl 8.9–10.1 mg/dL), phosphorus

J.P. Ingimarsson, MD
Department of Urology, Mayo College of Medicine, Mayo Clinic, Rochester, MN, USA
e-mail: Ingimarsson.Johann@mayo.edu

J.C. Lieske, MD (✉)
Division of Nephrology and Hypertension, Department of Internal Medicine, Mayo College of Medicine, Mayo Clinic, Rochester, MN, USA
e-mail: Lieske.John@mayo.edu

A.E. Kearns, R.A. Wermers (eds.), *Hyperparathyroidism: A Clinical Casebook*, DOI 10.1007/978-3-319-25880-5_3,
© Mayo Foundation for Medical Education and Research 2016

of 3.1 mg/dL (nl 2.5–4.5 mg/dL), and parathyroid hormone of 95 pg/mL (nl 15–65 pg/mL). Her 24-h urinary calcium was modestly elevated at 242 mg/day (normal for females <200 mg/day). Other notable values on the urine collection included a low volume (1200 mL) and a pH of 6.9 with a citrate of 419 mg/day (nl >430 mg/day). A subsequent sestamibi scan revealed an unequivocal left superior parathyroid adenoma.

Assessment and Diagnosis

Primary hyperparathyroidism (PHPT) is a known risk factor for urinary stone disease. Among patients presenting with urinary stone disease, the incidence of PHPT is 2–8 % [1]. In the era before routine serum calcium testing, 40–60 % of PHPT patients developed urinary calculi [2, 3]. In the current era, when more patients are diagnosed with asymptomatic PHPT based on blood calcium and parathyroid hormone (PTH) levels, most studies report a urinary stone incidence of less than 20 % [4]. This compares to a population urinary stone disease incidence of about 11 % [5]. On one extreme of the spectrum, among a cohort of patients with hypercalcemia, high PTH levels, and no secondary cause of hyperparathyroidism, Odvina and colleagues reported in 2007 that 60 % had a urinary stone [6]. In another cohort selected on the basis of surgically proven PHPT, Suh and colleagues reported in 2008 that renal sonograms revealed urinary stones in 7 % of asymptomatic patients [7].

The reason for increased lithogenesis in PHPT is still a matter of some uncertainty. Numerous studies have compared demographic factors as well as serum and urinary chemistries between PHPT patients with stones versus PHPT without stones, as well as controls. The best-established demographic risk factors are male gender and young age [8] (both unlike our current patient).

The physiologic actions of PTH supply some clues regarding possible mechanism(s) whereby PHPT might be associated with urinary stones. Major effects include stimulation of 1-alpha hydroxylation in the kidney, which in turn promotes formation of active 1,25-dihydroxy vitamin D, inhibition of renal phosphate reabsorption, and stimulation of bone resorption to release calcium and phosphate. Increased 1,25-dihydroxy vitamin D also stimulates gastrointestinal absorption of calcium and phosphorus. The net effect is to raise serum calcium but not phosphorus [9].

Although PTH also increases tubular reabsorption of calcium, net renal calcium excretion rises because the filtered load of calcium increases (due to the hypercalcemia) [10]. Since hypercalciuria is a well-defined risk factor for urinary stone disease, it is not surprising that PHPT might increase stone risk.

Nevertheless, the association between hypercalciuria and stone formation in patients with PHPT has been inconsistent in the literature. While some have found an association [6, 11–13], others find none [8, 14–16]. Thus a normal or relatively normal 24-h urine calcium excretion, as was the case for our patient, is often observed. It does seem that calcium metabolism is important, since calcium oxalate and phosphate stones predominate in PHPT, while uric acid stones are proportionally less common than in the general population [6, 10]. In addition, calcium phosphate stones appear to occur somewhat more commonly than in non-PHPT stone formers [10, 17]. Urine parameters other than calcium excretion have not been reproducibly associated with stone formation in PHPT. Polymorphisms in the calcium-sensing receptor gene may be associated with the risk of nephrolithiasis in PHPT [18].

Hypercalcemia is the most important clue to the diagnosis of PHPT in the setting of stone disease, since the vast majority of surgically proven cases will have at least some degree of elevation in serum calcium, often combined with hypophosphatemia [10]. Pooled from several studies, the mean serum calcium level for hyper parathyroid stone formers was

11.2 mg/dL (nl 8.9–10.1 mg/dL). A large portion of patients have values close to 10.5 mg/dL, which is the normal cutoff in many labs. Elevated serum calcium has a high positive prediction of hyperparathyroidism. The added feature of hypophosphatemia decreases the false-positive prediction. As PHPT is one of the few reversible causes of urinary stones, a high level of suspicion for the diagnosis is prudent in a stone former with even mild hypercalcemia [10, 19].

On the other hand, it is not possible to reliably diagnose PHPT in the absence of hypercalcemia, since in many such cases the elevation in PTH represents a physiologically appropriate response [9]. Thus routine screening of stone clinic populations with PTH levels in the absence of hypercalcemia is not recommended [19].

Management

The patient underwent an uneventful left superior parathyroidectomy. Unfortunately, 5 weeks later she suffered a myocardial infarct with somewhat a prolonged recovery. Therefore her asymptomatic renal stones were not addressed surgically at that time. Her serum calcium ranged from 8.7 to 9.7 mg/dL postoperatively.

Outcome

Fourteen and 31 months after the parathyroidectomy, the patient required surgery to remove ureteral stones. Their chemical composition was 80 % calcium oxalate monohydrate and 20 % hydroxyapatite. Prior to the latter event, she spontaneously passed a few other stones. In 8 years since the last stone surgery, she has not had a symptomatic stone event. A CT scan done for another indication 5 years after parathyroidectomy showed no further stones.

After parathyroidectomy hypercalciuria generally decreases [16, 20]. However, some studies have shown that in PHPT patients with prior stone history, the urinary calcium is more likely to remain above normal range and higher than in healthy controls [10, 15]. Further, serum phosphate remains in general lower in patients after parathyroidectomy for PHPT than in healthy controls [10].

The risk of nephrolithiasis decreases after a curative parathyroidectomy. However, the risk remains increased compared with the general population, with 16 % more stone events reported in post-parathyroidectomy patients than in the general population [21]. Of note patients with a prior history of stones and PHPT had 76 % more stone events than controls, whereas PHPT patients without prior stone history only had a 3 % higher risk than controls [21]. Another series reported a low risk (1.5 %) of renal stone recurrence among preoperative stone formers after parathyroidectomy and a much lower risk than observed in idiopathic stone formers (20 %) over the same time period [22].

With this in mind, the International Workshop on the Management of Asymptomatic PHPT in 2013 revised its recommendation taking a more assertive stand to state that imaging findings indicating calcium-containing stones in a patient with PHPT is an indication for parathyroidectomy [23].

While some of the stones passed after surgery may reflect those already formed at the time on parathyroidectomy, a third of patients will form one to four new stones per year in the first 5 years after parathyroidectomy [24]. Nevertheless most stone events happen in the first 4 years, and at 10 years the risk of kidney stone events is close to that of the general population [21].

Clinical Pearls/Pitfalls
- Renal stones are common in PHPT and are associated with younger age and male gender.
- PTH should be tested in stone formers with hypercalcemia.
- Among those with PHPT, a history of clinical stone events and/or the presence of radiologic stones is an indication for parathyroidectomy.
- Biochemical parameters before or after parathyroidectomy are not consistent predictors of renal stones.
- Renal stone risk decreases after parathyroidectomy, but probably remains elevated compared to the general population for up to 10 years.

Conflict of Interest All authors state that they have no conflicts of interest.

References

1. Rodman JS, Mahler RJ. Kidney stones as a manifestation of hypercalcemic disorders: hyperparathyroidism and sarcoidosis. Urol Clin North Am. 2000;27:275–85.
2. Pak CY, Nicar MJ, Peterson R, Zerwekh JE, Snyder W. A lack of unique pathophysiologic background for nephrolithiasis of primary hyperparathyroidism. J Clin Endocrinol Metab. 1981;53:536–42.
3. Broadus AE, Horst RL, Lang R, Littledike ET, Rasmussen H. The importance of circulating 1,25-dihydroxyvitamin D in the pathogenesis of hypercalciuria and renal-stone formation in primary hyperparathyroidism. N Engl J Med. 1980;302:421–6.
4. Rejnmark L, Vestergaard P, Mosekilde L. Nephrolithiasis and renal calcifications in primary hyperparathyroidism. J Clin Endocrinol Metab. 2011;96:2377–85.
5. Litwin MS, Saigal CS, editors. Urologic diseases in America. Table 9-2 urinary tract stones. US Department of Health and Human Services, Public Health Service, National Institutes of Health, National Institute of

Diabetes and Digestive and Kidney Diseases. Washington, DC: US Government Printing Office; 2012. p. 315. NIH Publication No. 12-7865.
6. Odvina CV, Sakhaee K, Heller HJ, Peterson RD, Poindexter JR, Padalino PK, Pak CY. Biochemical characterization of primary hyperparathyroidism with and without kidney stones. Urol Res. 2007;35:123–8.
7. Suh JM, Cronan JJ, Monchik JM. Primary hyperparathyroidism: is there an increased prevalence of renal stone disease? AJR Am J Roentgenol. 2008;191:908–11.
8. Elkoushy MA, Yu AX, Tabah R, Payne RJ, Dragomir A, Andonian S. Determinants of urolithiasis before and after parathyroidectomy in patients with primary hyperparathyroidism. Urology. 2014;84:22–6.
9. Kumar R, Thompson JR. The regulation of parathyroid hormone secretion and synthesis. J Am Soc Nephrol. 2011;22:216–24.
10. Parks JH, Coe FL, Evan AP, Worcester EM. Clinical and laboratory characteristics of calcium stone-formers with and without primary hyperparathyroidism. BJU Int. 2009;103:670–8.
11. Soreide JA, van Heerden JA, Grant CS, Lo CY, Ilstrup DM. Characteristics of patients surgically treated for primary hyperparathyroidism with and without renal stones. Surgery. 1996;120:1033–7.
12. Corbetta S, Baccarelli A, Aroldi A, Vicentini L, Fogazzi GB, Eller-Vainicher C, et al. Risk factors associated to kidney stones in primary hyperparathyroidism. J Endocrinol Invest. 2005;28:122–8.
13. Starup-Linde J, Waldhauer E, Rolighed L, Mosekilde L, Vestergaard P. Renal stones and calcifications in patients with primary hyperparathyroidism: associations with biochemical variables. Eur J Endocrinol. 2012;166:1093–100.
14. Silverberg SJ, Shane E, Jacobs TP, Siris ES, Gartenberg F, Seldin D, et al. Nephrolithiasis and bone involvement in primary hyperparathyroidism. Am J Med. 1990;89:327–34.
15. Frøkjaer VG, Mollerup CL. Primary hyperparathyroidism: renal calcium excretion in patients with and without renal stone disease before and after parathyroidectomy. World J Surg. 2002;26:532–5.
16. Berger AD, Wu W, Eisner BH, Cooperberg MR, Duh QY, Stoller ML. Patients with primary hyperparathyroidism—why do some form stones? J Urol. 2009;181:2141–5.
17. Pak CY, Poindexter JR, Adams-Huet B, Pearle MS. Predictive value of kidney stone composition in the detection of metabolic abnormalities. Am J Med. 2003;115:26–32.
18. Vezzoli G, Scillitani A, Corbetta S, Terranegra A, Dogliotti E, Guarnieri V, et al. Risk of nephrolithiasis in primary hyperparathyroidism is associated

with two polymorphisms of the calcium-sensing receptor gene. J Nephrol. 2015;28:67–72.

19. Pearle MS, Goldfarb DS, Assimos DG, Curhan G, Denu-Ciocca CJ, Matlaga BR, American Urological Assocation, et al. Medical management of kidney stones: AUA guideline. J Urol. 2014;192:316–24.

20. Rao DS, Phillips ER, Divine GW, Talpos GB. Randomized controlled clinical trial of surgery versus no surgery in patients with mild asymptomatic primary hyperparathyroidism. J Clin Endocrinol Metab. 2004;89:5415–22.

21. Mollerup CL, Vestergaard P, Frøkjaer VG, Mosekilde L, Christiansen P, Blichert-Toft M. Risk of renal stone events in primary hyperparathyroidism before and after parathyroid surgery: controlled retrospective follow up study. BMJ. 2002;325:807–10.

22. Rowlands C, Zyada A, Zouwail S, Joshi H, Stechman MJ, Scott-Coombes DM. Recurrent urolithiasis following parathyroidectomy for primary hyperparathyroidism. Ann R Coll Surg Engl. 2013;95:523–8.

23. Bilezikian JP, Brandi ML, Eastell R, et al. Guidelines for the management of asymptomatic primary hyperparathyroidism: summary statement from the fourth international workshop. J Clin Endocrinol Metab. 2014;99:3561–9.

24. Mollerup CL, Lindewald H. Renal stones and primary hyperparathyroidism: natural history of renal stone disease after successful parathyroidectomy. World J Surg. 1999;23:173–6.

Chapter 4
Primary Hyperparathyroidism and Osteoporosis

Naykky Singh Ospina and Daniel L. Hurley

Case Presentation

A 45-year-old premenopausal Caucasian woman presented to her primary care physician (PCP) for evaluation of atypical chest pain. During biochemical evaluation, she was found to have hypercalcemia (10.6 mg/dL, normal 8.9–10.1) associated with an elevated serum parathyroid hormone (PTH) value of 104 pg/mL (normal 15–65), consistent with primary hyperparathyroidism (PHPT).

She had no previous history of fractures and kidney stones or family history of hypercalcemia. Her calcium intake consisted of one cup of milk and one to two servings of cheese per day (estimated 500–600 mg/day). She was not taking calcium or vitamin D supplementation. Her only medication was sumatriptan for migraine headaches. Her general physical exam was normal.

Laboratory evaluation included a total 25-hydroxyvitamin D level of 27 ng/mL (optimal range 20–50), creatinine 0.7 mg/dL (normal 0.6–1.0), and 24-h urine calcium 300 mg (normal

N.S. Ospina, MD • D.L. Hurley, MD (✉)
Division of Endocrinology, Diabetes, Metabolism, and Nutrition,
Department of Internal Medicine, Mayo College of Medicine,
Mayo Clinic, Rochester, MN, USA
e-mail: singhospina.naykky@mayo.edu; hurley.daniel@mayo.edu

A.E. Kearns, R.A. Wermers (eds.), *Hyperparathyroidism:*
A Clinical Casebook, DOI 10.1007/978-3-319-25880-5_4,
© Mayo Foundation for Medical Education and Research 2016

<275). Dual energy x-ray absorptiometry (DXA) bone mineral density (BMD) was measured at the hips (total hip sites; left T score −1.2, right T score −1.0) and lumbar (L1–4) spine (T score −1.7).

A discussion of treatment options included parathyroidectomy versus observation, and the patient preferred medical observation.

Assessment and Diagnosis

PHPT has been associated with bone loss most notable in the cortical bone compared to cancellous bone [1, 2]. The prevalence of osteoporosis assessed by DXA in patients with PHPT has been found by Cipriani et al. to be close to 60 % with a prevalence of vertebral fracture of 35 % (study population with 91 % women and a mean age of 63 years) [3]. Conversely, the prevalence of PHPT in patients with osteoporosis has been reported between 0.5 and 6.1 % [4].

The identification of concomitant osteoporosis and PHPT is important since it may alter clinical management, as surgical correction of PHPT has been associated with improvement of BMD [5, 6].

Current clinical practice guidelines recommend DXA BMD evaluation in all patients with PHPT, as BMD results may change PHPT management toward surgery for potential skeletal benefits [5]. In a prospective study of patients with PHPT, only 14 % had a history of clinical fractures at baseline assessment but 60 % had osteoporosis based on DXA findings [3].

This DXA evaluation should include BMD measurement at the radius in addition to the spine and hips, as cortical (compact) bone is more susceptible than trabecular (cancellous) bone to the effects of PTH [2, 5].

The presence of osteoporosis (as defined by fragility fractures or a DXA T score ≤ -2.5) is a strong indication for surgical intervention in patients with PHPT. This recommendation is based on BMD improvement in patients that undergo surgical intervention [5, 7, 8].

In patients with PHPT who have a contraindication for surgery or who refuse surgical intervention, medical management is an alternative treatment [5, 9]. Most commonly, bisphosphonates are the treatment of choice based upon clinical studies showing improvement of BMD, although data regarding fracture outcomes are lacking [9]. A meta-analysis of patients with PHPT and calcium levels <12 mg/dL reported improved BMD at the lumbar spine and femoral neck in patients treated with surgery or bisphosphonates, without significant change in forearm BMD [7, 9]. In the studies that assessed BMD without PHPT intervention, decreased BMD was noted at the lumbar spine, femoral neck, and forearm at 2-year follow-up [7]. It is important to note that BMD change is only a surrogate marker for fracture outcome, for which clinical evidence is not available in patients with PHPT [7, 9].

There is no high-quality evidence available to be able to recommend when DXA BMD should be repeated after surgical intervention for PHPT. Studies have shown improvement in BMD between 12 and 36 months after surgical cure [10, 11]. A repeat BMD at 12–24-month follow-up is advised for patients who prefer observation or are receiving medical therapy [5].

Multiple localization techniques which help plan the surgical procedure are currently available. These studies should only be performed when surgery is a consideration, since the diagnosis of PHPT is based on biochemical evidence alone [5, 8].

Available localization techniques include neck ultrasound, sestamibi scintigraphy, computerized tomography (CT) scanning, magnetic resonance imaging (MRI), and catheter-based localization. Each of these modalities is associated with different advantages, disadvantages, costs and radiation dose. Overall, the sestamibi scan and neck ultrasound have sensitivities above 75 % and the four-dimensional CT (4D-CT) scan has a sensitivity of 89 %. The positive predictive value for each of these three techniques is above 90 % [12]. This highlights the point that the diagnosis of PHPT is a biochemical diagnosis. In addition, even when localization studies are used to help guide surgery, they might be negative in some cases.

There is a known relationship between dietary calcium intake and serum PTH levels that can have different effects on bone metabolism. There are concerns that reducing the calcium intake in patients with PHPT might lead to more pronounced stimulation of PTH secretion and a deleterious effect on bone; on the other hand, a reduced calcium intake might translate into decreased urinary calcium load and a lower risk of kidney stones [5]. A calcium food questionnaire study in 31 patients with asymptomatic PHPT found that calcium supplementation in subjects with a low dietary calcium intake (below 450 mg/day) resulted in a decrease in serum PTH (after 4 weeks) and improvement in BMD (at the end of 1-year follow-up) [13]. The present recommendation for calcium intake in patients with PHPT is the same as for patients without PHPT, due to lack of clinical evidence to the contrary [9, 13, 14].

Management

She received annual follow-up for 6 years by her primary care provider without any interim history for kidney stones, frac-

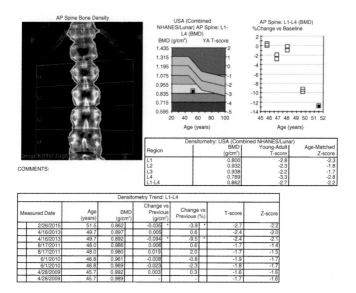

Fig. 4.1 Changes in lumbar spine BMD from baseline diagnosis of PHPT to before surgery 6 years later

tures, or worsening hypercalcemia. BMD during this time decreased at the lumbar spine by 13 % (*T* score −2.7) (Fig. 4.1), at the left hip by 5.6 % (*T* score −1.5), and at the right hip by 6.0 % (*T* score −1.4) (Fig. 4.2) with a significant decline in combined total hip BMD (Table 4.1). At her 6-year follow-up at age 51, she was referred for an endocrinology consultation. A right wrist BMD was also measured at this time and corresponded to a *T* score of −3.0 (Fig. 4.3). The potential benefits of surgical intervention to BMD and fracture risk were revisited, and a parathyroid scan (Fig. 4.4) was obtained prior to surgical evaluation.

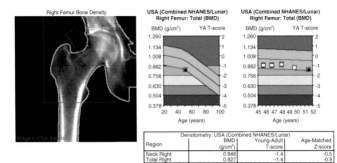

Fig. 4.2 Changes in right hip BMD from baseline diagnosis of PHPT to before surgery 6 years later

Table 4.1 Change in combined total hip bone mineral density (BMD) during follow up of primary hyperparathyroidism from baseline diagnosis to 6 years later

Combined total hip results:

 04/28/2009   BMD: 0.874 g/cm^2, T Score: -1.1
 06/01/2010   BMD: 0.872 g/cm^2, T Score: -1.1
 08/17/2011   BMD: 0.881 g/cm^2, T Score: -1.0
 04/16/2013   BMD: 0.838 g/cm^2, T Score: -1.3
 02/26/2015   BMD: 0.822 g/cm^2, T Score: -1.5

Change vs. Previous (2015–2013) difference: -0.016 g/cm^2 and -1.9 %

The least significant change (LSC) in BMD for the Total Hip is 0.036 g/cm^2

The absolute BMD change from previous (2013), 0.016 g/cm^2, is less than the LSC

The absolute BMD change from baseline (2009), 0.052 g/cm^2, is greater than the LSC

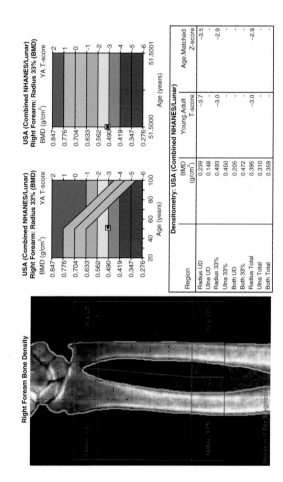

Right Forearm Bone Density

USA (Combined NHANES/Lunar)
Right Forearm: Radius 33% (BMD)

BMD (g/cm²)	YA T-score
0.847	2
0.776	1
0.704	0
0.633	-1
0.562	-2
0.490	-3
0.419	-4
0.347	-5
0.276	-6

Age (years) 20 40 60 80 100

USA (Combined NHANES/Lunar)
Right Forearm: Radius 33% (BMD)

BMD (g/cm²)	YA T-score
0.847	2
0.776	1
0.704	0
0.633	-1
0.562	-2
0.490	-3
0.419	-4
0.347	-5
0.276	-6

Age (years) 51.5000   51.5001

Densitometry: USA (Combined NHANES/Lunar)

Region	BMD (g/cm²)	Young.Adult T-score	Age.Matched Z-score
Radius UD	0.239	-3.7	-3.5
Ulna UD	0.148	-	-
Radius 33%	0.493	-3.0	-2.9
Ulna 33%	0.450	-	-
Both UD	0.205	-	-
Both 33%	0.472	-	-
Radius Total	0.395	-3.0	-2.9
Ulna Total	0.310	-	-
Both Total	0.359	-	-

Fig. 4.3 Right forearm BMD before surgery, consistent with the effects of PHPT on cortical bone

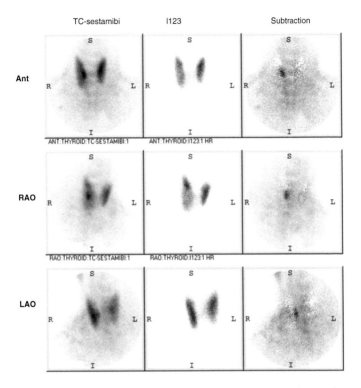

Fig. 4.4 Sestamibi scan showing intense right-sided neck uptake, consistent with a single parathyroid adenoma

Outcome

Minimally invasive parathyroidectomy was completed without complications, and she achieved surgical cure of her PHPT. Reassessment in 1 year with BMD measurement is planned to determine whether osteoporosis medications are necessary.

Clinical Pearls
- The diagnosis of PHPT is based on biochemical information and not on imaging studies. Although localization studies have a low false-negative rate, they should be performed only when surgery is a consideration, to help plan the surgical procedure.
- PHPT should be evaluated as a secondary cause of osteoporosis.
- Patients with PHPT should be screened for osteoporosis, as the presence of concomitant disease can impact clinical management.
- Surgical treatment is strongly recommended in patients with PHPT and osteoporosis. Medical treatment with bisphosphonates is an alternative option if surgery is contraindicated or refused.
- Patients with PHPT and osteoporosis should adhere to the Institute of Medicine recommendations regarding adequate intake of calcium and vitamin D (i.e., there is no need for calcium restriction).

Conflict of Interest All authors state that they have no conflicts of interest.

References

1. Khan A, Bilezikian J. Primary hyperparathyroidism: pathophysiology and impact on bone. CMAJ. 2000;163(2):184–7 [Review].
2. Silverberg SJ, Shane E, de la Cruz L, Dempster DW, Feldman F, Seldin D, et al. Skeletal disease in primary hyperparathyroidism. J Bone Miner Res. 1989;4(3):283–91 [Research Support, US Gov't, PHS].
3. Cipriani C, Biamonte F, Costa AG, Zhang C, Biondi P, Diacinti D, et al. Prevalence of kidney stones and vertebral fractures in primary hyperparathyroidism using imaging technology. J Clin Endocrinol Metab. 2015;100(4):1309–15 [Research Support, NIH, Extramural].

4. Bours SP, van den Bergh JP, van Geel TA, Geusens PP. Secondary osteoporosis and metabolic bone disease in patients 50 years and older with osteoporosis or with a recent clinical fracture: a clinical perspective. Curr Opin Rheumatol. 2014;26(4):430–9.

5. Bilezikian JP, Brandi ML, Eastell R, Silverberg SJ, Udelsman R, Marcocci C, et al. Guidelines for the management of asymptomatic primary hyperparathyroidism: summary statement from the Fourth International Workshop. J Clin Endocrinol Metab. 2014;99(10):3561–9 [Consensus Development Conference].

6. Cosman F, de Beur SJ, LeBoff MS, Lewiecki EM, Tanner B, Randall S, et al. Clinician's guide to prevention and treatment of osteoporosis. Osteoporos Int. 2014;25(10):2359–81.

7. Sankaran S, Gamble G, Bolland M, Reid IR, Grey A. Skeletal effects of interventions in mild primary hyperparathyroidism: a meta-analysis. J Clin Endocrinol Metab. 2010;95(4):1653–62 [Meta-Analysis Research Support, Non-US Gov't Review].

8. Udelsman R, Akerstrom G, Biagini C, Duh QY, Miccoli P, Niederle B, et al. The surgical management of asymptomatic primary hyperparathyroidism: proceedings of the Fourth International Workshop. J Clin Endocrinol Metab. 2014;99(10):3595–606 [Consensus Development Conference].

9. Marcocci C, Bollerslev J, Khan AA, Shoback DM. Medical management of primary hyperparathyroidism: proceedings of the fourth International Workshop on the Management of Asymptomatic Primary Hyperparathyroidism. J Clin Endocrinol Metab. 2014;99(10):3607–18 [Consensus Development Conference].

10. Dy BM, Grant CS, Wermers RA, Kearns AE, Huebner M, Harmsen WS, et al. Changes in bone mineral density after surgical intervention for primary hyperparathyroidism. Surgery. 2012;152(6):1051–8.

11. Rolighed L, Vestergaard P, Heickendorff L, Sikjaer T, Rejnmark L, Mosekilde L, et al. BMD improvements after operation for primary hyperparathyroidism. Langenbecks Arch Surg. 2013;398(1):113–20.

12. Kunstman JW, Kirsch JD, Mahajan A, Udelsman R. Clinical review: parathyroid localization and implications for clinical management. J Clin Endocrinol Metab. 2013;98(3):902–12 [Review].

13. Jorde R, Szumlas K, Haug E, Sundsfjord J. The effects of calcium supplementation to patients with primary hyperparathyroidism and a low calcium intake. Eur J Nutr. 2002;41(6):258–63 [Clinical Trial Randomized Controlled Trial].

14. Ross AC, Manson JE, Abrams SA, Aloia JF, Brannon PM, Clinton SK, et al. The 2011 report on dietary reference intakes for calcium and vitamin D from the Institute of Medicine: what clinicians need to know. J Clin Endocrinol Metab. 2011;96(1):53–8.

Chapter 5
Parathyroid Hormone Measurement Considerations in Primary Hyperparathyroidism

Robert A. Wermers and Stefan K. Grebe

Case Presentation

A 48 year-old female was referred by oncology to endocrinology for evaluation of hypercalcemia. She was premenopausal at the time of her diagnosis of stage 1 (T1c, N0, M0) invasive ductal carcinoma breast cancer 5 years ago. The tumor cells were estrogen receptor negative, progesterone receptor positive, and HER2/neu negative. Treatment had consisted of wide local excision after initial breast conservation surgery which showed high-grade ductal carcinoma in situ (DCIS) at one of the margins with a single sentinel lymph node negative for metastatic disease, followed by radiation, adjuvant chemotherapy, and

R.A. Wermers, MD (✉)
Division of Endocrinology, Diabetes, Metabolism, and Nutrition,
Department of Internal Medicine, Mayo College of Medicine,
Mayo Clinic, Rochester, MN, USA
e-mail: wermers.robert@mayo.edu

S.K. Grebe, MD, PhD
Department of Laboratory Medicine and Pathology, Mayo College of
Medicine, Mayo Clinic, Rochester, MN, USA
e-mail: grebe.stefan@mayo.edu

A.E. Kearns, R.A. Wermers (eds.), *Hyperparathyroidism:*
A Clinical Casebook, DOI 10.1007/978-3-319-25880-5_5,
© Mayo Foundation for Medical Education and Research 2016

subsequent tamoxifen therapy. Due to side effects with tamoxifen combined with menopausal transition, she was switched to aromatase inhibitor therapy 2 years after her initial diagnosis. She had remained without evidence of breast cancer recurrence based on her mammogram, laboratory testing, and oncology history and physical examination. However, hypercalcemia was identified a year prior to referral, with a serum calcium of 10.3 mg/dL (nl, 8.9–10.1). Her maximum serum calcium level was 11.1 mg/dL which led to her referral. Her repeat laboratory tests were as follows: serum calcium, 10.4 mg/dL; PTH, 30 pg/ mL (nl, 15–50 pg/mL); phosphorus, 4 mg/dL (nl, 2.5–4.5); albumin, 4.0 g/dL (nl, 3.5–5.0); 25-hydroxyvitamin D, 31 ng/mL; and 24 h urine calcium, 152 mg (20–275 mg/specimen). All of the following labs were normal: TSH, complete blood count, creatinine, AST, and alkaline phosphatase.

She denied history of nephrolithiasis, fragility fractures, polyuria, polydipsia, abdominal pain, fatigue, and constipation. Due to a declining dual-energy X-ray absorptiometry (DXA) bone mineral density (BMD) since initiating aromatase inhibitor therapy (femur neck T-score of −0.5 and lumbar spine T-score of −0.9), she was started on risedronate 1 year prior to her referral. Her family history was devoid of hypercalcemia or any other familial endocrine syndromes, and she denied prior head or neck radiation. Her dietary calcium intake was estimated at 600–800 mg/day, and she did not take calcium or vitamin D supplements and had never used lithium or hydrochlorothiazide. Her medications at referral were metoprolol tartrate, venlafaxine, anastrozole, levothyroxine, and risedronate. Her physical examination was unremarkable.

Assessment and Diagnosis

Primary hyperparathyroidism (PHPT) is defined by hypercalcemia associated with an elevated or non-suppressed serum

PTH measured by a two-site immunometric assay with high specificity for intact PTH (full-length PTH, PTH(1-84)). Such an assay is superior to C-terminal and mid-molecule PTH assays in distinguishing PHPT from non-PTH-mediated causes of hypercalcemia. Hypercalcemia of malignancy and other non-PTH-mediated hypercalcemic processes typically present with a low-serum intact PTH concentration [1], whereas intact PTH levels are reported to be elevated in approximately 80 % of patients with PHPT [2]. In hypercalcemic patients with PTH concentrations that are not elevated above the healthy population reference interval, levels in the upper one-half to one-third of the reference interval are considered inappropriately "normal" and have been used as a cutoff for PHPT [3]. However, PTH levels in the lower third of the reference interval have also been observed in an estimated 3 % of cases of pathologically confirmed cases of PHPT [4–7].

Lower than expected PTH measurements can be caused by a several biological factors. PTH in PHPT is influenced by the dynamic nature of its secretion [8], its circadian rhythm [9], the serum calcium level [10], vitamin D stores [11], and calcium intake [12]. Hemoconcentration, immobilization, and pH-dependent changes in protein-bound calcium can also influence both PTH and calcium measurements [13].

Other considerations in case of unexpectedly low PTH measurements center on assay-specific problems. Extremely high serum PTH concentrations can result in a hook effect in single-step, sandwich-type immunometric assays. In this type of assay, the assay's capture and detection antibodies are present at the same time to interact with the patient sample. When the PTH concentration in a sample exceeds the combined molar concentration of detection and capture antibody, each of these antibodies will be individually saturated with PTH, and very few actual sandwiches of AB-PTH-AB can be formed. This results in a false-low PTH measurement [7]. Serial sample dilution is required to obtain the true PTH concentration. Atypical, but bioactive, forms of PTH might also be encountered and are often not detected by PTH assays [7]. The presence of such variants might be suspected, if serial sample dilutions deviate significantly from linearity [7].

Immunometric assays in general, including PTH assays, might also be vulnerable to false low interference that is exerted by chemicals or biomolecules that interfere with the assay's chemistry, analyte capture, or signal detection. General interferences of this nature include an extremely high lipid or protein content of a sample, both of which can hinder binding of the analyte to the assay antibodies, or high concentrations of optically active substances, like bilirubin or hemoglobin, which can interfere with signal detection. In addition, depending on an assay's precise configuration, there may be other interferences that can cause false low results in one or another (but not every) assay system. Examples of these include high biotin levels or anti-streptavidin antibodies in a patient serum [14–16]. Many assays use biotin-streptavidin binding to capture the antibody onto a solid support before signal readout from the detection antibody. Excess biotin or anti-streptavidin antibodies in a patient sample will prevent this reaction, leading to false low interference in assays using biotin-streptavidin capture. Antibodies or chemicals in a patient's serum that interfere with components of the signal generation system can similarly cause false low results. Individually, the rates of biological interferences, PTH concentration/fragment-dependent interferences, and assay-related interferences are very low, but collectively, these problems occur with appreciable, though still relatively low, frequency.

In our case, none of these interferences appeared to be present, and given the lower than expected PTH and the patient's history of breast cancer, further evaluation of non-PTH-mediated causes of PHPT was performed, all the while bearing in mind that the most likely diagnosis was still PHPT. Indeed, PHPT has been described when coexistent causes of hypercalcemia, including malignancy, have also been present [17]. Further testing in this patient revealed the following: 1,25-dihydroxyvitamin D at 21 pg/mL (nl, 22–67) and PTH-related peptide (PTHrP) at 110 pmol/L (nl, <2). Assessment for complications related to PHPT was also performed. Her kidney-ureter-bladder (KUB) plain film radiograph with tomography was negative for kidney stones, and her one-third radius DXA BMD T-score was 0.7. Because of the unexpected PTHrP result, the test was repeated and the laboratory was called. The repeat PTHrP was 95 pmol/L and the specimen had linear dilution. Subsequently, a bone scan and fluorodeoxyglucose (FDG) positron emission tomography (PET) scan were performed. Both were unremarkable.

Management

A further repeat PTHrP was performed at a different reference laboratory and was undetectable. Both PTHrP assays used goat antibodies but had different binding sites. Subsequently, the specimen was reanalyzed at the initial laboratory after pretreatment of the sample with heterophile-blocking reagents, with no change in the elevated result. However, a repeat dilution series was nonlinear, consistent with interference from either a heterophile antibody or the presence of PTHrP fragments or variants.

Based on the patient's relatively stable and mild hypercalcemia, heterophile (from the Greek words heteros meaning the other, and philos meaning the friend – friend of the other) antibodies (HAB) were felt to be the most likely culprit. HAB are endogenous antibodies found in serum or plasma of patients that can bind to immunoglobulins of other species, such as the antibodies used as reagents for immunoassays [18]. They primarily affect two-site immunoassays, where they lead to false-positive results in >80 % of cases, by bridging detection and capture antibody in the absence of analyte (Fig. 5.1). Occasionally, when HAB only bind to either capture or detection antibody, they can also cause a false low result. HAB fall into three major groups: (i) polyspecific antibodies, as are often seen after viral infections, which bind a variety of targets, including sometimes assays antibodies; these antibodies are common in the population (up to 30 % prevalence at any given time),

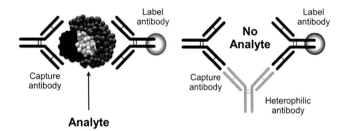

Fig. 5.1 Two-site immunoassay with bridging of two antibodies with antigen (*left*) and heterophile antibodies bridging the two antibodies (*right*) independent of the antigen, resulting in an increase in the bound-labeled antibody concentration

but rarely cause assay problems, because they have relatively low avidity to most assay antibodies; (ii) antibodies directed at species-conserved components of immunoglobulins; the prime example of this group is rheumatoid factor, which is an antibody against the Fc portion of immunoglobulins; these HAB are much less common than the polyspecific HAB, but because of their higher avidity to assay antibodies, they are more likely to cause problems; and (iii) high-affinity/avidity and high-titer antibodies that are specifically directed against mouse, rabbit, or goat IgG (common species for assay antibodies); these antibodies are rare; they require the patient to be specifically sensitized to mouse, rabbit, or goat (animal handling or diagnostic/therapeutic use of ABs) – but account for most HAB interferences. Cancer patients may be more likely than the general population to have interfering HAB [19].

In retrospect, it was clear that this patient did not have cancer-associated hypercalcemia, and perhaps, further testing was not needed in this regard. The positive PTHrP results should probably have been flagged as a "red herring" from the outset. The patient's history of hypercalcemia was too long and the hypercalcemia is too mild to be consistent with cancer-associated hypercalcemia, which is usually a preterminal event (median time to death of 30 days) that is associated with rapidly progressive, severe, and symptomatic hypercalcemia [20].

Outcome

The patient was reassured that she likely had mild, uncomplicated PHPT as what was observed. One year later, she continued to have stable, mild hypercalcemia and remained asymptomatic.

Clinical Pearls/Pitfalls
- The clinical and natural history of PHPT is very important when interpreting calcium biomarker laboratory results.
- PTH levels in PHPT are generally above the midpoint of the healthy population reference interval.
- Consider repeating PTH when the diagnosis of PHPT is unclear, especially since dynamic changes in calcium metabolism may occur in the presence of secondary contributing factors or if there is suspicion of assay interference.
- Consider additional non-PTH-mediated causes of hypercalcemia when the PTH is lower than expected for a diagnosis of PHPT.
- If repeat PTH measurement remains inappropriately in the lower half of the normal range despite continued hypercalcemia and other causes of hypercalcemia are not present, then serial sample dilution may be considered.
- When considering malignancy-related hypercalcemia, be mindful that a positive PTHrP result only has a high positive predictive value if the pretest probability for tumor-related hypercalcemia is high, i.e., when the patient has obvious progressive cancer and a short history of severe, progressive, and symptomatic hypercalcemia.
- Understand the laboratory assays you order and communicate with your laboratory if unexpected results are encountered.

Conflict of Interest All authors state that they have no conflicts of interest.

References

1. Kao PC, van Heerden JA, Grant CS, Klee GG, Khosla S. Clinical performance of parathyroid hormone immunometric assays. Mayo Clin Proc. 1992;67:637–45.
2. Glendenning P, Gutteridge DH, Retallack RW, Stuckey BG, Kermode DG, Kent GN. High prevalence of normal total calcium and intact PTH in 60 patients with proven primary hyperparathyroidism: a challenge to current diagnostic criteria. Aust NZ J Med. 1998;28:173–8.
3. Lundgren E, Rastad J, Thrufjell E, Akerstrom G, Ljunghall S. Population-based screening for primary hyperparathyroidism with serum calcium and parathyroid hormone values in menopausal women. Surgery. 1997;121:287–94.
4. Glendenning P, Pullan PT, Gulland D, Edis AJ. Surgically proven primary hyperparathyroidism with a suppressed intact parathyroid hormone. Med J Aust. 1996;165:197–8.
5. Hollenberg AN, Arnold A. Hypercalcemia with low-normal serum intact PTH: a novel presentation of primary hyperparathyroidism. Am J Med. 1991;91:547–8.
6. Khoo TK, Baker CH, Abu-Lebdeh HS, Wermers RA. Suppressibility of parathyroid hormone in primary hyperparathyroidism. Endocr Pract. 2007;13:785–9.
7. Lafferty FW, Hamlin CR, Corrado KR, Arnold A, Shuck JM. Primary hyperparathyroidism with a low-normal, atypical serum parathyroid hormone as shown by discordant immunoassay curves. J Clin Endocrinol Metab. 2006;91:3826–9.
8. Samuels MH, Veldhuis J, Cawley C, et al. Pulsatile secretion of parathyroid hormone in normal young subjects: assessment by deconvolution analysis. J Clin Endocrinol Metab. 1993;77:399–403.
9. Calvo MS, Eastell R, Offord KP, Bergstralh EJ, Burritt MF. Circadian variation in ionized calcium and intact parathyroid hormone: evidence for sex differences in calcium homeostasis. J Clin Endocrinol Metab. 1991;72:69–76.
10. Khosla S, Ebeling PR, Firek AF, Burritt MM, Kao PC, Heath 3rd H. Calcium infusion suggests a "set-point" abnormality of parathyroid gland function in familial benign hypercalcemia and more complex disturbances in primary hyperparathyroidism. J Clin Endocrinol Metab. 1993;76:715–20.

11. Grey A, Lucas J, Horne A, Gamble G, Davidson JS, Reid IR. Vitamin D repletion in patients with primary hyperparathyroidism and coexistent vitamin D insufficiency. J Clin Endocrinol Metab. 2005;90:2122–6.

12. Tohme JF, Bilezikian JP, Clemens TL, Silverberg SJ, Shane E, Lindsay R. Suppression of parathyroid hormone secretion with oral calcium in normal subjects and patients with primary hyperparathyroidism. J Clin Endocrinol Metab. 1990;70:951–6.

13. Heath 3rd H. Postural and venous stasis-induced changes in total calcium. Mayo Clin Proc. 2005;80:1101.

14. Waghray A, Milas M, Nyalakonda K, Siperstein AE. Falsely low parathyroid hormone secondary to biotin interference: a case series. Endocr Pract. 2013;19:451–5.

15. Meany DL, de Beur SM J, Bill MJ, Sokoll LJ. A case of renal osteodystrophy with unexpected serum intact parathyroid hormone concentrations. Clin Chem. 2009;55:1737–9.

16. Rulander NJ, Cardamone D, Senior M, Snyder PJ, Master SR. Interference from anti-streptavidin antibody. Arch Pathol Lab Med. 2013;137:1141–6.

17. Gallacher SJ, Fraser WD, Farquharson MA, et al. Coincidental occurrence of primary hyperparathyroidism and cancer-associated hypercalcaemia in a middle-aged man. Clin Endocrinol (Oxf). 1993;38:433–7.

18. Bolstad N, Warren DJ, Nustad K. Heterophilic antibody interference in immunometric assays. Best Pract Res Clin Endocrinol Metab. 2013;27:647–61.

19. Preissner CM, O'Kane DJ, Singh RJ, Morris JC, Grebe SK. Phantoms in the assay tube: heterophile antibody interferences in serum thyroglobulin assays. J Clin Endocrinol Metab. 2003;88:3069–74.

20. Ralston SH, Gallacher SJ, Patel U, Campbell J, Boyle IT. Cancer-associated hypercalcemia: morbidity and mortality. Clinical experience in 126 treated patients. Ann Intern Med. 1990;112:499–504.

Chapter 6
Parathyroidectomy Outcomes and Pathology in Primary Hyperparathyroidism

Robert A. Wermers and Lori A. Erickson

Case Presentation

A 59 year-old female was referred for evaluation of primary hyperparathyroidism (PHPT). She had enjoyed excellent health her entire life, but during a routine health screen was found to have a serum calcium of 10.7 mg/dL (nl, 8.9–10.1). A repeat calcium once again was elevated at 10.6 mg/dL with a PTH that was 2 ½-fold times the upper limit of normal. Subsequent review of her prior laboratory work revealed that her calcium was slightly elevated 9 years prior and was high normal after that measurement. She denied symptoms related to hypercalcemia such as involuntary weight loss, abdominal pain, polyuria,

R.A. Wermers, MD (✉)
Division of Endocrinology, Diabetes, Metabolism, and Nutrition,
Department of Internal Medicine, Mayo College of Medicine,
Mayo Clinic, Rochester, MN, USA
e-mail: wermers.robert@mayo.edu

L.A. Erickson, MD
Department of Laboratory Medicine and Pathology,
Mayo College of Medicine, Mayo Clinic, Rochester, MN, USA
e-mail: Erickson.Lori@mayo.edu

A.E. Kearns, R.A. Wermers (eds.), *Hyperparathyroidism:
A Clinical Casebook*, DOI 10.1007/978-3-319-25880-5_6,
© Mayo Foundation for Medical Education and Research 2016

fatigue, or depression and did not have a history of nephrolithiasis or fragility fractures. Her past medical history was significant for hypertension that was well controlled with an ACE inhibitor, thiazide diuretic, and a beta-blocker. She was on estrogen replacement therapy after a hysterectomy for benign disease. She also had primary hypothyroidism and was on stable levothyroxine therapy. Her family history was unremarkable for familial hypercalcemia. Her physical examination was unremarkable.

Assessment and Diagnosis

The patient's lab work is consistent with PHPT. Although she is on a thiazide diuretic which has been associated with hypercalcemia, most patients with thiazide-associated hypercalcemia have underlying PHPT, and her higher PTH level would be consistent with PHPT in this context [1]. After a diagnosis of PHPT, clinical assessment for related complications may include dual-energy X-ray absorptiometry bone mineral density of the spine, hip, and nondominant wrist and imaging for nephrolithiasis by computed tomography (CT) of the abdomen and pelvis without contrast, renal ultrasound, or kidney-ureter-bladder (KUB) plain film radiographs with tomography. This patient had a KUB with tomography that revealed small opaque renal calculi in both kidneys. Hence, she was referred to endocrine surgery for consideration of parathyroidectomy. A 24-h urine calcium and creatinine is often assessed if surgery is a consideration due to the possibility of familial hypocalciuric hypercalcemia (FHH). However, her negative family history for PHPT or hypercalcemia combined with normal serum calcium levels on prior measurements essentially rules out FHH as the cause of her hypercalcemia. Patients with FHH are also usually devoid of PHPT complications (e.g., nephrolithiasis), and PTH levels are elevated in only 5–25 % of FHH subjects [2, 3].

Localization of the parathyroid pathology is often considered once a decision is made to proceed with surgery. Although there are several modalities utilized for parathyroid localization [4], the decision regarding which test to use is often determined by the test which has the highest sensitivity and specificity at the institution performing the study. This patient underwent a parathyroid scan with I-123 and 99mTc sestamibi which revealed a right inferior parathyroid adenoma.

Management

The patient underwent uncomplicated cervical exploration where in the right inferior position in the thyrothymic tongue a 350 mg parathyroid adenoma was identified and excised.

Outcome

Her postoperative calcium dropped to 9.4 mg/dL. Pathology revealed a 370 mg, $1.1 \times 0.8 \times 0.6$ cm parathyroid lipoadenoma (Fig. 6.1). Complications related to parathyroid surgery are rare but most commonly include recurrent laryngeal nerve injury (0.5–1 %), hematoma formation (0.2 %), and hypocalcemia (0.1 %) [5]. Disease cure depends on the parathyroidectomy surgical volume, but in highly experience centers, >95 % of patients are normocalcemic postoperatively [5]. PTH on the other hand remains elevated in 8–40 % of patients with normocalcemia after parathyroidectomy for unclear reasons [6]. However, most of these patients do not get recurrent hypercalcemia (i.e., recurrent PHPT) [7]. Persistent PHPT is defined by failure of biochemical cure with the initial parathyroid surgery. Recurrent PHPT is defined by an initial biochemical cure (normocalcemia), followed by recurrent disease >6 months after the initial surgery.

Parathyroid glands typically weigh 20–40 mg, while those weighing more than 50–60 mg are usually abnormal [8]. Normal parathyroid glands consist of chief cells – the main source of PTH, transitional cells, oxyphil cells, and adipose tissue. Adipose tissue is the primary component of the parathyroid stroma and occupies approximately 20–30 % of an adult parathyroid gland. Also parathyroid cellularity can be highly variable within a single gland, among glands in the same patient, and between patients. It also varies by age, sex, and body habitus, among others.

PHPT is due to a single parathyroid adenoma in 80–85 % or more of patients [9]. Chief cell parathyroid adenomas are the most common pathologic variant in PHPT [10]. Oxyphil cells typically comprise less than 5 % of parathyroid volume [11], but oxyphil parathyroid adenomas can be seen in PHPT and have been associated with larger adenomas [12–14]. However, a recent case-matched study found no significant difference in weight between oxyphil and chief cell adenomas [15].

PHPT due to parathyroid lipoadenomas are rare but, clinically, present in a similar fashion to those associated with common parathyroid pathologic variants [16]. Parathyroid lipoadenomas are defined by extensive stromal adipose tissue, myxoid change, and fibrosis [17]. Clear cell parathyroid adenomas are composed of cells with finely vacuolated cytoplasm in a solid or acinar pattern [18]. Atypical parathyroid adenomas have atypical features such as mitoses and fibrous bands but lack definitive invasion or metastases. They generally behave in a benign fashion [19].

A definitive histopathological diagnosis of parathyroid carcinoma is difficult and often presents as severe PHPT where it is suspected or as PHPT recurrence 2–3 years after the initial parathyroid surgery. Classical pathologic criteria include uniform sheets of cells arranged in a lobular pattern separated by dense fibrous trabeculae, mitotic figures in tumors cells, and capsular

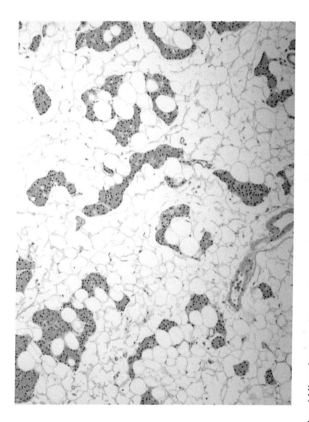

Fig. 6.1 Parathyroid lipoadenoma with proliferation of parenchymal parathyroid tissue and stromal elements with adipose tissue comprising greater than 50 % of the adenoma. The parenchymal tissue is comprised of oxyphilic cells and small numbers of chief cells organized in small groups and thin, branching cords. Hematoxylin and Eosin stain: medium power

and vascular invasion [20, 21]. Invasive growth is required for a diagnosis of parathyroid carcinoma. Only 3–30 % of patients have evidence of regional lymph node involvement or distant metastases at the initial surgery (see Chap. 10) [22]. Parathyromatosis is a rare pathologic variant in PHPT that is characterized by small nodules of hyperplastic parathyroid tissue composed primarily of chief cells that are scattered throughout the soft tissues of the neck and upper mediastinum [19, 23]. Clinically, this condition is characterized by recurrent or persistent PHPT. On occasion, parathyroid glands removed in patients with prior thyroidectomy or re-explorative parathyroid surgery may present challenges to the surgeon and pathologist due to fibrosis (see Chap. 11).

PHPT due to parathyroid hyperplasia, which accounts for approximately 15 % of PHPT, is defined as multiple parathyroid glands with proliferation of parenchymal cells leading to parathyroid gland enlargement independent of secondary factors that stimulate PTH production. Preoperative imaging studies and intraoperative PTH monitoring aid in differentiating single from multiple gland disease. Chief cell hyperplasia is the most common form of parathyroid hyperplasia, but rarely clear cell hyperplasia and lipohyperplasia are seen. Asymmetric hyperplasia is a challenging issue as only around 50 % of PHPT has symmetric enlargement of all four glands. Approximately one-third of PHPT hyperplasia is due to familial parathyroid disorders (e.g., MEN, MEN2A, MEN4, hyperparathyroidism-jaw tumor syndrome, familial isolated PHPT).

Clinical Pearls/Pitfalls
- After the diagnosis of PHPT is confirmed, evaluate for related complications.
- Parathyroidectomy has a high rate of cure and complications are rare.

- Review the outcome of parathyroid surgery, utilizing serum calcium rather than PTH for surveillance postoperatively.
- Parathyroid adenomas are the cause of PHPT in ≥80 % of patients and pathologically are usually due to chief cell adenomas, but oxyphil adenomas, lipoadenomas, clear cell adenomas, and atypical parathyroid adenomas are additional pathologic variants.
- Parathyroid carcinoma often presents with severe PHPT or is identified with disease recurrence 2–3 years after the initial parathyroid surgery.
- Parathyroid hyperplasia is the cause of PHPT in approximately 15 % of patients and is seen in familial parathyroid disorders such as MEN1, MEN2A, MEN4, hyperparathyroidism-jaw tumor syndrome, and familial isolated PHPT.

Conflict of Interest All authors state that they have no conflicts of interest.

References

1. Wermers RA, Kearns AE, Jenkins GD, Melton 3rd LJ. Incidence and clinical spectrum of thiazide-associated hypercalcemia. Am J Med. 2007;120:911 e919–915.
2. Christensen SE, Nissen PH, Vestergaard P, Mosekilde L. Familial hypocalciuric hypercalcaemia: a review. Curr Opin Endocrinol Diabetes Obes. 2011;18:359–70.
3. Arnold A, Marx SJ. Familial primary hyperparathyroidism (Including MEN, FHH, and HPT-JT). In: Primer on the metabolic bone diseases and disorders of mineral metabolism. 8th ed. Ames: Wiley; 2013. p. 553–61.

4. Kunstman JW, Kirsch JD, Mahajan A, Udelsman R. Clinical review: parathyroid localization and implications for clinical management. J Clin Endocrinol Metab. 2013;98:902–12.

5. Udelsman R, Lin Z, Donovan P. The superiority of minimally invasive parathyroidectomy based on 1650 consecutive patients with primary hyperparathyroidism. Ann Surg. 2011;253:585–91.

6. Pathak PR, Holden SE, Schaefer SC, Leverson G, Chen H, Sippel RS. Elevated parathyroid hormone after parathyroidectomy delays symptom improvement. J Surg Res. 2014;190:119–25.

7. Carsello CB, Yen TW, Wang TS. Persistent elevation in serum parathyroid hormone levels in normocalcemic patients after parathyroidectomy: does it matter? Surgery. 2012;152:575–81; discussion 581–3.

8. Erickson LA. Atlas of endocrine pathology. New York: Springer; 2014. p. 103.

9. Rosai J DR, Carcangiu ML, Frable WJ, Tallini G. Tumors of the thyroid and parathyroid glands (AFIP atlas of tumor pathology: series 4). American Registry of Pathology, Silver Spring, MD (Maryland); 2015, p. 513.

10. Bedetti CD, Dekker A, Watson CG. Functioning oxyphil cell adenoma of the parathyroid gland: a clinicopathologic study of ten patients with hyperparathyroidism. Hum Pathol. 1984;15:1121–6.

11. Akerstrom G, Rudberg C, Grimelius L, et al. Histologic parathyroid abnormalities in an autopsy series. Hum Pathol. 1986;17:520–7.

12. Erickson LA, Jin L, Papotti M, Lloyd RV. Oxyphil parathyroid carcinomas: a clinicopathologic and immunohistochemical study of 10 cases. Am J Surg Pathol. 2002;26:344–9.

13. Fleischer J, Becker C, Hamele-Bena D, Breen TL, Silverberg SJ. Oxyphil parathyroid adenoma: a malignant presentation of a benign disease. J Clin Endocrinol Metab. 2004;89:5948–51.

14. Giorgadze T, Stratton B, Baloch ZW, Livolsi VA. Oncocytic parathyroid adenoma: problem in cytological diagnosis. Diagn Cytopathol. 2004;31:276–80.

15. Howson PKS, Aniss A, Pennington T, Gill AJ, Dodds T, Delbridge LW, Sidhu SB, Sywak MS. Oxyphil cell parathyroid adenomas causing primary hyperparathyroidism: a clinico-pathological correlation. Endocr Pathol. 2015;26:250–4.

16. Chow LS, Erickson LA, Abu-Lebdeh HS, Wermers RA. Parathyroid lipoadenomas: a rare cause of primary hyperparathyroidism. Endocr Pract. 2006;12:131–6.

17. Abul-Haj SK, Conklin H, Hewitt WC. Functioning lipoadenoma of the parathyroid gland. Report of a unique case. N Engl J Med. 1962; 266:121–3.

18. Rosai J DR, Carcangiu ML, Frable WJ, Tallini G. Tumors of the thyroid and parathyroid glands (AFIP atlas of tumor pathology: series 4). American Registry of Pathology Silver Spring, MD (Maryland); 2015. p. 532.
19. Fernandez-Ranvier GG, Khanafshar E, Jensen K, et al. Parathyroid carcinoma, atypical parathyroid adenoma, or parathyromatosis? Cancer. 2007;110:255–64.
20. Bondeson L, Sandelin K, Grimelius L. Histopathological variables and DNA cytometry in parathyroid carcinoma. Am J Surg Pathol. 1993;17:820–9.
21. Schantz A, Castleman B. Parathyroid carcinoma. A study of 70 cases. Cancer. 1973;31:600–5.
22. Marcocci C, Cetani F, Rubin MR, Silverberg SJ, Pinchera A, Bilezikian JP. Parathyroid carcinoma. J Bone Miner Res. 2008;23:1869–80.
23. Lentsch EJ, Withrow KP, Ackermann D, Bumpous JM. Parathyromatosis and recurrent hyperparathyroidism. Arch Otolaryngol Head Neck Surg. 2003;129:894–6.

Chapter 7
Localization Considerations in Persistent Primary Hyperparathyroidism

Robert A. Wermers and Geoffrey B. Thompson

Case Presentation

A 42-year-old female was referred for evaluation of persistent primary hyperparathyroidism (PHPT). Her history was significant for continued lithium use for over 10 years. Prior to diagnosis she had a syncopal episode, where evaluation revealed a serum calcium of 13.6 mg/dL. Her parathyroid hormone (PTH) level was several fold elevated on multiple measures at 200–350 pg/mL. She had associated symptoms including increased thirst, polyuria, nausea, cognitive decline, and a 35-lb weight loss. A preoperative parathyroid scan, neck ultrasound, and neck computed tomography (CT) scan were non-localizing.

R.A. Wermers, MD (✉)
Division of Endocrinology, Diabetes, Metabolism, and Nutrition,
Department of Internal Medicine, Mayo College of Medicine,
Mayo Clinic, Rochester, MN, USA
e-mail: wermers.robert@mayo.edu

G.B. Thompson, MD
Department of Surgery, Mayo College of Medicine, Mayo College of Medicine, Mayo Clinic, Rochester, MN, USA
e-mail: thompson.geoffrey@mayo.edu

A.E. Kearns, R.A. Wermers (eds.), *Hyperparathyroidism:*   57
A Clinical Casebook, DOI 10.1007/978-3-319-25880-5_7,
© Mayo Foundation for Medical Education and Research 2016

She underwent a 5-h parathyroid exploration which included excision of her right and left superior parathyroid glands, biopsy of a normal right inferior parathyroid, and a left upper thymectomy. Her intraoperative PTH did not change, and postoperatively, her calcium remained 11–13 mg/dL. She denied use of hydrochlorothiazide and calcium supplements and was on cholecalciferol 2000 IU daily in addition to cinacalcet 60 mg twice daily started after surgery. She did not have knowledge of her family's medical history and denied a history of head or neck radiation.

Her current lab work on cinacalcet included a serum calcium 12.7 mg/dL (nl, 8.9–10.1), phosphorus 2.1 mg/dL (nl, 2.5–4.5), normal creatinine, albumin 4.4 g/dL (nl, 3.5–5.0), PTH 194 pg/mL (nl, 15–65), and 24-h urine calcium 204 mg/dL with a fractional excretion of filtered calcium of 0.02. A repeat parathyroid scan suggested a possible left inferior parathyroid adenoma on the combination of single-photon emission computed tomography (SPECT) and computed tomography (CT) images (SPECT/CT). Neck ultrasound showed a 4×6×9 mm oval hypoechoic nodule deep to the left common carotid artery more suggestive of a lymph node that was biopsied and had a PTH washout of <20 pg/mL. A four-dimensional computed tomography (4D CT) showed no definite parathyroid adenoma, but anterior to the aortic arch and to the right of midline, there was a 7-mm nodule with mild early arterial enhancement with washout on delayed imaging (Fig. 7.1).

Assessment and Diagnosis

Persistent PHPT presents several diagnostic considerations including the possibility of an ectopic parathyroid adenoma, parathyroid carcinoma, multigland parathyroid disease, and familial benign hypocalciuric hypercalcemia (FHH). FHH is an

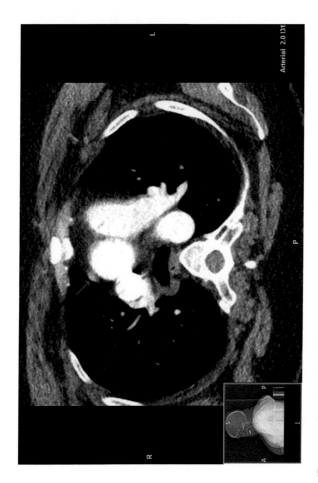

Fig. 7.1 4D computed tomography (CT) parathyroid scan demonstrating a 7-mm nodule with mild early arterial enhancement in the upper mediastinum, anterior to the aortic arch and to the right of midline (*arrow*). No abnormality in this location was identified on nuclear medicine imaging. No other suspicious lesions to suggest an ectopic parathyroid adenoma were seen

autosomal dominant disorder with a nearly 100 % penetrance of hypercalcemia at all ages caused by an inactivating mutation of the *CASR* gene, which encodes the calcium-sensing receptor [1–3]. Patients with FHH are generally devoid of complications seen in PHPT such as nephrolithiasis, and their risk of osteoporosis is similar to that expected in the general population. Also, serum PTH levels are elevated in only 5–25 % of FHH subjects [3, 4]. Renal calcium clearance to creatinine clearance below 0.01 is suggestive of FHH, and in this case, the fractional excretion of filtered calcium of 0.02 is not consistent with this diagnosis. In this patient, it is important to consider that lithium use over several years can lead to parathyroid gland hyperplasia [5–8]. Lithium-associated hyperparathyroidism is more common in younger females (mean age 41 years) than patients with classical PHPT [8].

Reoperation for persistent PHPT is an expensive procedure with an estimated cost of $5711 [9, 10]. More recent estimates based on Center for Medicare and Medicaid Service (CMS) clinical fee schedule amounts for parathyroidectomy indicate higher costs than this in 2013. The increased cost of reoperation emphasizes the importance of utilizing an experienced parathyroid surgeon with high cure rates. Given the increased risk of complications during reoperation for persistent PHPT, some have suggested that the costs of reoperation are more than twice that the cost of initial surgery [11]. Indeed, increased parathyroid surgery volume has been associated with decreased complication rates and improved postsurgical outcomes [12, 13].

In this case, consultation was obtained from an experience endocrine surgeon. It was determined that re-exploration without more defining localization put the patient at an increased risk for unsuccessful surgery. Importantly the parathyroid scan and neck ultrasound with fine-needle aspiration (FNA) of left inferior neck lesion were not consistent with a parathyroid adenoma. PTH washout levels, when positive, are a median of

3963 pg/mL (results >100 pg/mL PTH level considered posi-tive) in our experience and are useful for distinguishing parathy-roid lesions from thyroid or lymphatic tissue [14].

4D CT is a multiphasic, cross-sectional imaging study that captures the rapid uptake and washout of contrast from parathy-roid adenomas [15] and has been shown to be useful in the reoperative setting [16, 17] and in patients with non-localizable disease on sestamibi or ultrasonography [18]. There is an increase in total radiation dose (10.4 mSv) with 4D CT and it is less readily available [15]. Although there was a 7-mm nodule anterior to the aortic arch on the 4D CT, more precise confirma-tion of an ectopic mediastinal adenoma would be recommended prior to considering thoracic surgery. Hence, in this case, the next best strategy would be to proceed with venous PTH sampling.

Management

The patient underwent parathyroid venous sampling after stop-ping cinacalcet, which revealed a PTH of >3000 pg/mL from the thymic vein compared to 9–150 pg/mL from other sites, consis-tent with a mediastinal parathyroid adenoma. Selective PTH venous sampling (SVS) is generally reserved for patients with recurrent or persistent hyperparathyroidism with nondiagnostic radiologic localization studies. Serial samples for PTH are obtained from the superior vena cava and bilateral brachioce-phalic, internal jugular, vertebral, thymic, superior, middle, and inferior thyroid veins. In reoperative cases SVS has a reported sensitivity of 71–90 % [15]. As in this patient, a combination of localization modalities is often utilized and complementary to each other in localizing the diseased parathyroid gland(s) in patients with persistent or recurrent PHPT.

Outcome

The patient proceeded with a right thoracoscopy with excision of an anterior ectopic parathyroid adenoma. Her intraoperative PTH dropped from a baseline of 161 pg/mL to 13.6 pg/ml at 20 min after removal. Her serum calcium and phosphorus normalized postoperatively.

Clinical Pearls/Pitfalls
- Selection of an experienced endocrine surgeon is important in successful parathyroidectomy outcomes.
- Persistent or recurrent PHPT presents several diagnostic considerations including an ectopic parathyroid adenoma, parathyroid carcinoma, multigland parathyroid disease, and FHH.
- Prior to consider reoperation in persistent or recurrent PHPT, preoperative localization is important and often requires a combination of localization modalities including a parathyroid scan, neck ultrasound, 4D CT, FNA of suspected parathyroid lesions with PTH washout, and SVS.

Conflicts of Interest All authors state that they have no conflicts of interest.

References

1. Law Jr WM, Heath 3rd H. Familial benign hypercalcemia (hypocalciuric hypercalcemia). Clinical and pathogenetic studies in 21 families. Ann Intern Med. 1985;102:511–9.
2. Marx SJ, Attie MF, Levine MA, Spiegel AM, Downs Jr RW, Lasker RD. The hypocalciuric or benign variant of familial hypercalcemia: clinical and biochemical features in fifteen kindreds. Medicine (Baltimore). 1981;60:397–412.

3. Arnold A, Marx SJ. Familial primary hyperparathyroidism (Including MEN, FHH, and HPT-JT). In: Primer on the metabolic bone diseases and disorders of mineral metabolism. 8th ed. Ames: Wiley; 2013:553–61.
4. Christensen SE, Nissen PH, Vestergaard P, Mosekilde L. Familial hypocalciuric hypercalcaemia: a review. Curr Opin Endocrinol Diabetes Obes. 2011;18:359–70.
5. Larkins RG. Lithium and hypercalcaemia. Aust N Z J Med. 1991;21:675–7.
6. Mallette LE, Eichhorn E. Effects of lithium carbonate on human calcium metabolism. Arch Intern Med. 1986;146:770–6.
7. Mallette LE, Khouri K, Zengotita H, Hollis BW, Malini S. Lithium treatment increases intact and midregion parathyroid hormone and parathyroid volume. J Clin Endocrinol Metab. 1989;68:654–60.
8. McHenry CR, Lee K. Lithium therapy and disorders of the parathyroid glands. Endocr Pract. 1996;2:103–9.
9. Morris LF, Zanocco K, Ituarte PH, et al. The value of intraoperative parathyroid hormone monitoring in localized primary hyperparathyroidism: a cost analysis. Ann Surg Oncol. 2010;17:679–85.
10. Sosa JA, Powe NR, Levine MA, Bowman HM, Zeiger MA, Udelsman R. Cost implications of different surgical management strategies for primary hyperparathyroidism. Surgery. 1998;124:1028–35; discussion 1035–6.
11. Doherty GM, Weber B, Norton JA. Cost of unsuccessful surgery for primary hyperparathyroidism. Surgery. 1994;116:954–7; discussion 957–8.
12. Mitchell J, Milas M, Barbosa G, Sutton J, Berber E, Siperstein A. Avoidable reoperations for thyroid and parathyroid surgery: effect of hospital volume. Surgery. 2008;144:899–906; discussion 906–7.
13. Stavrakis AI, Ituarte PH, Ko CY, Yeh MW. Surgeon volume as a predictor of outcomes in inpatient and outpatient endocrine surgery. Surgery. 2007;142:887–99; discussion 887–9.
14. Bancos I, Grant CS, Nadeem S, et al. Risks and benefits of parathyroid fine-needle aspiration with parathyroid hormone washout. Endocr Pract. 2012;18:441–9.
15. Kunstman JW, Kirsch JD, Mahajan A, Udelsman R. Clinical review: parathyroid localization and implications for clinical management. J Clin Endocrinol Metab. 2013;98:902–12.
16. Mortenson MM, Evans DB, Lee JE, et al. Parathyroid exploration in the reoperative neck: improved preoperative localization with 4D-computed tomography. J Am Coll Surg. 2008;206:888–95; discussion 895–6.
17. Rodgers SE, Hunter GJ, Hamberg LM, et al. Improved preoperative planning for directed parathyroidectomy with 4-dimensional computed tomography. Surgery. 2006;140:932–40; discussion 940–1.
18. Day KM, Elsayed M, Beland MD, Monchik JM. The utility of 4-dimensional computed tomography for preoperative localization of primary hyperparathyroidism in patients not localized by sestamibi or ultrasonography. Surgery. 2015;157:534–9.

Chapter 8
Ectopic Parathyroid Adenoma

Jad G. Sfeir and Matthew T. Drake

Case Presentation

A 50-year-old female was diagnosed with primary hyperpara-thyroidism (PHPT) based on a laboratory evaluation obtained during evaluation for recurrent nephrolithiasis. She described a history that included passing greater than 300 calcium oxalate kidney stones over the course of the past 20 years despite medical therapy with hydrochlorothiazide and potassium citrate, as well as maintenance of a low oxalate diet. Laboratory evaluation over time had revealed a progressive mild increase in serum calcium and parathyroid hormone (PTH) levels. Her most recent values are listed in Table 8.1. ^{99m}Tc-sestamibi/iodine-123 scintigraphy demonstrated a discordant focus of activity in the superior mediastinum consistent with an ectopic parathyroid adenoma, with no evidence for a thyroidal location (Fig. 8.1).

J.G. Sfeir, MD • M.T. Drake, MD, PhD (✉)
Division of Endocrinology, Diabetes, Metabolism, and Nutrition,
Department of Internal Medicine, Mayo College of Medicine,
Mayo Clinic, Rochester, MN, USA
e-mail: jgsfeir@gmail.com; drake.matthew@mayo.edu

A.E. Kearns, R.A. Wermers (eds.), *Hyperparathyroidism:*
A Clinical Casebook, DOI 10.1007/978-3-319-25880-5_8,
© Mayo Foundation for Medical Education and Research 2016

65

Assessment and Diagnosis

The incidence of ectopic parathyroid glands in patients with PHPT has been reported to range from 5 % to 20 % [1–5]. Ectopic parathyroid glands can significantly impact morbidity and clinical outcomes primarily due to failure during parathyroid exploration and subsequent requirement for reoperation. It has been estimated that 24–53 % of cases of reoperation for persistent or recurrent PHPT are due to the ectopic location of the diseased gland(s) [2, 6, 7].

The clinical and biochemical features of orthotopic versus ectopic parathyroid adenomas have been evaluated in several cohorts. On average, ectopic parathyroid adenomas are both usually significantly larger and associated with higher serum calcium levels [1, 4, 8]. In one cohort, it was also noted that radiographic evidence of osteitis fibrosa cystica was more frequent in patients with ectopic parathyroid adenomas [1]. There do not appear to be other significant differences in terms of patient characteristics (age, gender) or biochemical (serum phosphorus and PTH levels), clinical (presence of nephrolithiasis, hypertension, pancreatitis, and osteoporosis), or histopathologic features (adenoma, hyperplasia, or carcinoma) in subjects with orthotopic versus ectopic parathyroid adenomas.

The parathyroid glands originate from the third and fourth pharyngeal pouches, with differentiation beginning during the fifth and sixth weeks of development. Whereas parathyroid

Table 8.1 Patient's most recent laboratory data

Analyte	Results	Reference range
Calcium	10.5	8.9–10.1 mg/dL
Parathyroid hormone (PTH)	68	15–65 pg/mL
Creatinine	0.8	0.6–1.1 mg/dL
25-hydroxyvitamin D	31	20–50 ng/mL
24-h urine calcium excretion	439	25–300 mg/24 h

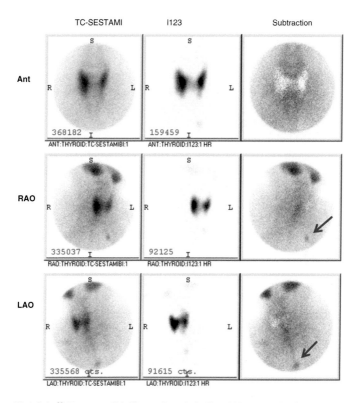

Fig. 8.1 ⁹⁹ᵐTc-sestamibi (first column); iodine-123 (second column) and subtraction (third column) scintigraphy images showing a discordant focus of activity in the superior mediastinum consistent with an ectopic parathyroid adenoma. *Ant* anterior, *RAO* right anterior oblique, *LAO* left anterior oblique

tissue from the fourth pharyngeal pouch eventually migrates to give rise to the superior parathyroid glands, parathyroid tissue from the third pharyngeal pouch migrates caudally before arresting at the level of the thyroid to become the inferior parathyroid glands. Due to their longer migration path, the inferior parathyroid glands have a greater probability of becoming ecto-pic [9]. Notably, inferior glands commonly have associated thymic tissue due to the common third pharyngeal pouch embryonic origin of the thymus and inferior parathyroid glands. The most common locations for ectopic inferior parathyroid glands are intrathymic, the anterosuperior mediastinum, intra-thyroidal, associated with the thyrothymic ligament, or in the submandibular area (Fig. 8.2). Less commonly, ectopic parathy-roid glands derived from the inferior parathyroid can be found in the aortopulmonary window or associated with the pericar-dium, hypopharynx, nasopharynx, vagus nerve sheath, or poste-rior cervical triangle [1, 3–5, 10–12]. Superior parathyroid glands, when ectopic, are most commonly localized to the tra-cheoesophageal groove, retroesophageal space, posterosuperior mediastinum, intrathyroidal, carotid sheath, or paraesophageal space. One potential explanation for the ectopy of superior glands is that with disease development the parathyroid gland becomes larger and heavier, leading to vertical displacement by gravity [1, 3, 4, 10, 13].

Surgical and autopsy data demonstrate that most ectopic parathyroid glands originate from inferior glands (62 % vs. 38 % from superior glands) [4]. Most are accessible via a cervi-cal incision due to tracheoesophageal groove (28–43 %), intra-thymic (24–31 %), or intrathyroidal (7–22 %) locations. The remainder are most frequently mediastinal (14–26 %) or located in the carotid sheath (7–9 %), aortopulmonary window, or sub-maxillary region [1, 2, 4]. In a cohort of mediastinal ectopic parathyroid glands performed at the Mayo Clinic, 45 % of patients required open thoracotomy or mediastinotomy, while 55 % of patients underwent a minimally invasive approach (such as video-assisted thoracoscopy, manubrium split, or tran-scervical approach) [18]. No significant difference in outcomes over a mean 3-year follow-up period was seen between subjects who underwent open versus minimally invasive surgical approaches.

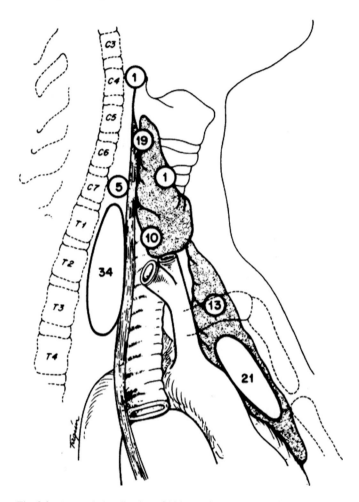

Fig. 8.2 Anatomic localization of 104 ectopic parathyroid glands. Superior posterior mediastinum ($n=34$); anterior mediastinum ($n=21$); dorsum of the upper ($n=19$) and lower ($n=10$) poles of the thyroid; within the thymic tongue ($n=13$); retroesophageal ($n=5$); at the angle of the jaw ($n=1$); and intrathyroidal ($n=1$) (Reprinted from Wang et al. [10] with permission)

Most surgeries performed for ectopic parathyroid gland resection are reoperations due to recurrent or persistent hyperparathyroidism disease after initial surgery. Reoperations typically occur in referral tertiary care centers. Due to the complexity of these operations and the potential for significant scar tissue present after initial extended parathyroid gland explorations, identifying an experienced parathyroid surgeon can be as essential as detecting the diseased parathyroid gland.

In the absence of preoperative localization, the surgeon typically carefully inspects all four orthotopic parathyroid glands in order to detect any abnormal gland. When less than four glands are found, it is recommended that the surgeon carefully inspects likely ectopic locations accessible via a cervical approach including the tracheoesophageal groove, thymus, ipsilateral thyroid, and upper cervical region [13].

Multiple imaging modalities are available for parathyroid adenoma localization and are associated with varying degrees of localization accuracy. Most reported cohorts, although limited in terms of sample sizes, suggest that patients are more likely to undergo successful surgical resection if localizing techniques are employed preoperatively [6]. Furthermore, preoperative localization for identification of ectopic glands can alter the operative approach depending on the ectopic gland location (i.e., substernal, aortopulmonary, or submandibular locations) [4, 10, 14].

Protocols for imaging prior to initial surgery are center specific and are typically based on local data in large referral tertiary care centers. However, prior to reoperation for persistent or recurrent PHPT, most surgical centers perform some combination of preoperative and/or intraoperative localization techniques (including intraoperative PTH measurements, intraoperative gamma probe, or a frozen section of the removed surgical specimen) [7, 15].

[99m]Tc-sestamibi scintigraphy has the highest sensitivity of localizing a single adenoma (90 %). The sensitivity, however, is decreased for double adenomas (30–73 %) and hyperplasia (45–60 %). Combining ^{99m}Tc-sestamibi scintigraphy with ^{123}I or

^{99m}Tc/^{99m}Tc-sestamibi subtraction eliminates potential false-positive results from thyroid nodules [13]. In one series, the positive predictive value for the detection of ectopic glands was 100 % compared to 98 % for parathyroid glands in normal anatomic locations [4]. On rare occasions, false negatives may result from ectopic parathyroid adenomas located at the carotid bifurcation as this location can sometimes be mistaken for physiological activity of the ipsilateral submandibular gland [16]. For completeness, scintigraphy should extend from the base of the jaw to the base of the heart in order to detect any ectopic glands along the full embryologic migratory course of the inferior glands [17].

Combination with another imaging technique can at times improve accuracy of preoperative localization. As example, intrathymic and aortopulmonary adenomas may have similar mediastinal activity on ^{99m}Tc-sestamibi scintigraphy. Oblique or lateral images might help in differentiating these two locations. Single-photon emission computed tomography (SPECT) allows for determination of depth relative to the thyroid gland [17], with Doppman et al. suggesting that SPECT imaging be considered whenever ^{99m}Tc-sestamibi scintigraphy demonstrates a deep mediastinal adenoma [12]. Alternatively, in some cases additional computed tomography (CT) or magnetic resonance imaging (MRI) may provide additional valuable information for the surgeon. Both CT and MRI have demonstrated great ability to detect ectopic parathyroid glands. Importantly, although CT is more readily available, it may have comparatively lower definition within the thyroid area [13].

Management

In addition to the parathyroid scan with ^{99m}Tc-sestamibi/iodine-123 scintigraphy, the patient had SPECT/CT images of the neck and chest which confirmed the ectopic location of her parathyroid adenoma. In conjunction with an experienced endocrine surgeon, a thoracic surgery team with significant previous experience in minimally invasive ectopic mediastinal parathyroid gland excision [18] evaluated the patient. After consultation, both surgical teams agreed that a left thoracoscopic approach was indicated. The endocrine surgeon was present during the surgery and assisted in intraoperative identification of the ectopic gland.

Outcome

The patient underwent resection of the mediastinal ectopic parathyroid adenoma identified on preoperative imaging via a left thoracoscopic approach. Pathology confirmed a 430-mg parathyroid adenoma. Intraoperative PTH measurements confirmed cure after the resection of the adenoma based on a decline from a baseline value of 74 to 24 pg/mL at 20 min following resection. Postoperative biochemical testing revealed serum calcium 9.2 mg/dL, ionized calcium 5.17 mg/dL (nl, 4.80–5.70 mg/dL), and PTH 55 pg/mL.

Clinical Pearls/Pitfalls

- Referral to a tertiary medical center with an experienced parathyroid surgeon and a radiology service with expertise in parathyroid imaging is important in patients in whom an ectopic parathyroid adenoma is suspected.
- Ectopic adenomas are usually significantly larger and associated with higher serum calcium levels compared to orthotopic adenomas.

- When less than four glands are identified intraoperatively, it is recommended that the surgeon carefully inspects common ectopic locations accessible via a cervical approach.
- Prior to reoperation for persistent or recurrent PHPT, most referral tertiary care centers perform some combination of preoperative and/or intraoperative localization techniques.
- Extending scintigraphy from the base of the jaw to the base of the heart allows for detection of ectopic inferior glands.
- Combining scintigraphy with another imaging technique, such as SPECT, CT, or MRI, can at times improve accuracy of preoperative localization.

Conflicts of Interest All authors state that they have no conflicts of interest.

References

1. Mendoza V, Ramírez C, Espinoza AE, González GA, Peña JF, Ramírez ME, et al. Characteristics of ectopic parathyroid glands in 145 cases of primary hyperparathyroidism. Endocr Pract. 2010;16(6):977–81.
2. Shen W, Düren M, Morita E, et al. Reoperation for persistent or recurrent primary hyperparathyroidism [with discussion]. Arch Surg. 1996;131:861–9.
3. Kaplan EL, Yashiro T, Salti G. Primary hyperparathyroidism in the 1990s: choice of surgical procedures for this disease. Ann Surg. 1992;215(4):300–17.
4. Phitayakorn R, McHenry CR. Incidence and location of ectopic abnormal parathyroid glands. Am J Surg. 2006;191(3):418–22; discussion 422–3.

5. Arnault V, Beaulieu A, Lifante JC, Sitges Serra A, Sebag F, Mathonnet M, et al. Multicenter study of 19 aortopulmonary window parathyroid tumors: the challenge of embryologic origin. World J Surg. 2010;34(9):2211–6.

6. Bagul A, Patel HP, Chadwick D, Harrison BJ, Balasubramanian SP. Primary hyperparathyroidism: an analysis of failure of parathyroidectomy. World J Surg. 2014;38(3):534–41.

7. Nawrot I, Chudziński W, Ciąćka T, Barczyński M, Szmidt J. Reoperations for persistent or recurrent primary hyperparathyroidism: results of a retrospective cohort study at a tertiary referral center. Med Sci Monit. 2014;20:1604–12.

8. Thompson NW, Eckhauser FE, Harness JK. The anatomy of primary hyperparathyroidism. Surgery. 1982;92:814–21.

9. Young WF. The Netter collection of medical illustrations. 2nd ed. Philadelphia: Elsevier; 2011.

10. Wang CA. Parathyroid re-exploration. A clinical and pathological study of 112 cases. Ann Surg. 1977;186(2):140–5.

11. Jaskowiak N, Norton JA, Alexander HR, Doppman JL, Shawker T, Skarulis M, et al. A prospective trial evaluating a standard approach to reoperation for missed parathyroid adenoma. Ann Surg. 1996;224(3):308–20.

12. Doppman JL, Skarulis MC, Chen CC, Chang R, Pass HI, Fraker DL, et al. Parathyroid adenomas in the aortopulmonary window. Radiology. 1996;201(2):456–62.

13. Gouveia S, Rodrigues D, Barros L, Ribeiro C, Albuquerque A, Costa G, Carvalheiro M. Persistent primary hyperparathyroidism: an uncommon location for an ectopic gland – case report and review. Arq Bras Endocrinol Metabol. 2012;56(6):393–403.

14. Billingsley KG, Fraker DL, Doppman JL, et al. Localization and operative management of undescended parathyroid adenomas in patients with persistent primary hyperparathyroidism. Surgery. 1994;116:982–90.

15. Daliakopoulos SI, Chatzoulis G, Lampridis S, Pantelidou V, Zografos O, Ioannidis K, et al. Gamma probe-assisted excision of an ectopic parathyroid adenoma located within the thymus: case report and review of the literature. J Cardiothorac Surg. 2014;9:62.

16. Axelrod D, Sisson JC, Cho K, et al. Appearance of ectopic undescended inferior parathyroid adenomas on technetium-99m-sestamibi scintigraphy. Arch Surg. 2003;138:1214–8.

17. Smith JR, Oates ME. Radionuclide imaging of the parathyroid glands: patterns, pearls, and pitfalls. Radiographics. 2004;24(4):1101–15.

18. Said SM, Cassivi SD, Allen MS, Deschamps C, Nichols 3rd FC, Shen KR, Wigle DA. Minimally invasive resection for mediastinal ectopic parathyroid glands. Ann Thorac Surg. 2013;96(4):1229–33.

Chapter 9
Parathyroid Surgery in Multiple Endocrine Neoplasia Type 1

T.K. Pandian, EeeLN H. Buckarma, and David R. Farley

Case Presentation

A 19-year-old female known to be part of a family with multiple endocrine neoplasia type 1 (MEN-1) and identified MENIN protein mutation initially presented with neuroglycopenia. Her medical workup revealed masses in the pancreas. She ultimately underwent a distal pancreatectomy with enucleation of the pancreatic head lesions for multiple insulinomas. Prior to that operation, her serum calcium was noted to be 10.8 mg/dL (nl, 8.9–10.1), and the parathyroid hormone (PTH) level was 68 pg/mL (nl, 15–65). She had no symptoms or non-laboratory signs of primary hyperparathyroidism (PHPT) at that time.

Shortly after her pancreatic surgery, she developed severe and persistent nausea. Despite a thorough medical evaluation, no organic intra-abdominal cause was found for her symptomatology. Six weeks after her pancreatic surgery, her

T.K. Pandian, MD, MPH • E.H. Buckarma, MD • D.R. Farley, MD (✉)
Department of Surgery, Mayo College of Medicine, Mayo Clinic,
Rochester, MN, USA
e-mail: pandian.twinkle@mayo.edu; buckarma.eeeln@mayo.edu;
farley.david@mayo.edu

A.E. Kearns, R.A. Wermers (eds.), *Hyperparathyroidism:*
A Clinical Casebook, DOI 10.1007/978-3-319-25880-5_9,
© Mayo Foundation for Medical Education and Research 2016

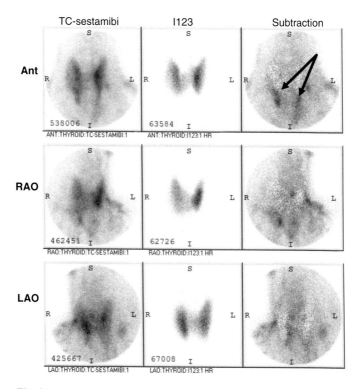

serum calcium was noted to be 11.6 ng/dL and the PTH was
78 pg/mL. A trial of cinacalcet (a calcimimetic agent acting
on chief cells in parathyroid glands to lower PTH secretion
and subsequently serum calcium levels) was undertaken and
her nausea immediately resolved. Given her laboratory findings suggestive of PHPT, a sestamibi localization scan was
obtained (Fig. 9.1).

Fig. 9.1 Nuclear medicine parathyroid single-photon emission computed
tomography (SPECT) revealing increased sestamibi uptake in the inferior
thyroid lobes bilaterally (*arrows*)

Assessment and Diagnosis

The classical medical mnemonic of the "3 Ps" identifies the pancreas, pituitary, and parathyroid glands as the major organ systems affected in MEN-1. Among these, PHPT is the most common manifestation and occurs in 88–97 % of MEN-1 patients [1]. In contrast, only 4–5 % of patients with sporadic PHPT are subsequently diagnosed with MEN-1 [2]. PHPT is usually the initial clinical feature found in patients with MEN-1 and typically presents by the third or fourth decade of life [1, 3]. Current international guidelines recommend annual assessment of serum calcium and PTH levels in known MEN-1 patients as a screening measure [4].

Asymmetric, multi-gland parathyroid disease is the norm in these individuals [3, 5–7], and therefore, management can be more complex than in patients with sporadic, single-gland PHPT. In the past, the multi-gland nature of PHPT in MEN-1 was thought to be due to circulating humoral factors that led to diffuse parathyroid hyperplasia [8, 9]. This belief has shifted over the years, and it is currently believed that parathyroid growth in MEN-1 is a neoplastic process which results in the development of multiple parathyroid adenomas [1, 5, 8]. Based on this multi-gland nature, preoperative imaging for adenoma localization is rarely indicated and of limited benefit [4].

The main treatment for PHPT in MEN-1 is surgical removal of hyperfunctioning glands. Eliminating PHPT in these patients will reduce the risk of nephrolithiasis and fractures and has been shown to improve quality of life [3]. Individuals with concurrent gastrinoma have even been found to have reduced gastrin levels after parathyroidectomy due to lower serum calcium levels [10]. The optimal surgical strategy for parathyroidectomy in MEN-1 patients remains controversial [1, 3, 6, 11–13].

Surgical options include subtotal parathyroidectomy (sub-PTX; removal of 3 or, more commonly, 3.5 parathyroid glands) or total parathyroidectomy (totPTX) with autotransplantation. Most experienced endocrine surgeons would also suggest that a transcervical thymectomy be included with any parathyroid operation in patients with MEN-1 [7, 14–16]. Both subPTX and totPTX have inherent challenges and are best performed by experienced parathyroid surgeons. The major risk for subPTX is recurrent or persistent hyperparathyroidism and is reported to occur in 16–54 % of patients within 5–10 years after surgery [1, 7, 12]. Leaving a small remnant (<40 mg) of normal-appearing parathyroid tissue is optimal, but with a disorder named "Multiple Endocrine Neoplasia," it is no surprise that recurrent PHPT may occur over years of follow-up as the remnant enlarges. Total parathyroidectomy with autotransplantation on the other hand may lead to permanent hypocalcemia in up to 30 % of patients [12, 17]. A completely aparathyroid state is unnatural and requires dutiful calcium supplementation with careful medical follow-up. Conversely, some MEN-1 patients with transplanted parathyroid tissue may actually develop recurrent PHPT as the transplanted tissue enlarges over time.

In a 2011 systematic review and meta-analysis, Shreinemakers and colleagues assessed the optimal surgical approach for PHPT in MEN-1 patients. Based on their own experience at a single center and 12 additional studies over a 42-year period, they found that patients undergoing anything less than subPTX (i.e., one- or two-gland parathyroidectomy) had a significantly higher risk of developing recurrent and persistent PHPT compared to subPTX or totPTX (OR 3.11, 95 % CI 2.00–4.84) [3]. Those that underwent subPTX were then compared to totPTX patients; there were no major differences in rates of recurrent and persistent PHPT between these two groups. Patients who received subPTX did, however, have a lower risk of permanent hypoparathyroidism (OR 0.25, 95 % CI 0.11–0.54) [3]. Based on this work, the authors preferred the use of sub-PTX in MEN-1 patients over all other surgical options. A more recent randomized-controlled trial involving 17 patients with sub-PTX vs. 15 patients with totPTX and parathyroid autotransplantation suggests there are no differences between these two approaches when performed by experienced surgeons in a standardized fashion [15]. The authors note, however, that the totPTX group had a longer aparathyroid state while the autografts regained function.

Based on this literature and our own long-term experience with MEN-1 patients, our practice relies on (1) bilateral neck exploration, (2) visualization of four or more parathyroid glands, (3) cervical thymectomy, (4) removal of 3.5 parathyroid glands (subPTX), and (5) consideration for parathyroid auto-transplantation (into strap muscles or subcutaneous fat of the upper chest) if the remaining remnant's blood supply is threatened. All four parathyroids should be identified and assessed for abnormality before any are resected. The smallest and most normal-looking gland (gross appearance) is utilized for the remaining remnant; it is ideal if it is an inferior gland and tacked to the trachea away from the recurrent laryngeal nerve. We prefer this approach for most patients with MEN-1 undergoing initial surgery for PHPT. Preoperative imaging for localization is occasionally utilized in very young patients.

Management

Our patient underwent subPTX with full four-gland exploration, cervical thymectomy, and three-gland parathyroidectomy (left inferior [230 mg], right inferior [830 mg], and right superior gland [380 mg]). The left superior gland (visually appeared to be normal and less than 40 mg in size) was left intact on its viable blood supply. Her intraoperative PTH decreased from a baseline of 62.6 to 23 pg/mL at 10-min post-excision. Her PTH was 15 pg/mL on postoperative day number 1.

Seven years after her parathyroidectomy, the patient began to have symptoms of nausea, similar to what she experienced immediately after her pancreas surgery. No organic intra-abdominal cause was found. Laboratory studies revealed a serum calcium of 11.1 mg/mL. The PTH was found to be 58 pg/mL.

Etiologies for recurrent PHPT include heterogeneity in gland size at the index operation leading to insufficient resection [18], supernumerary or ectopic glands missed during the initial surgery, [6], and the progressive neoplastic potential inherent to remaining parathyroid tissue in MEN-1 patients [7]. The treatment for this frustrating situation in these patients is complicated and varies based on the surgical experience of each institution and surgeon, and especially the previous surgical intervention(s).

Options include reoperation, percutaneous alcohol ablation (PetA), and medical therapies. Success rates for reoperation in MEN-1 are highly variable [3, 7, 12, 16, 19], but reoperation does portend a greater risk for recurrent laryngeal nerve injury [3, 7, 16]. Unpublished data from our institution reveal that after the 2nd (or more) operation(s) for recurrent pHPT in patients with MEN-1, only 35 % are normocalcemic at 1-year follow-up. The use of PetA in the event of recurrence has been described with initial normocalcemia in 50–82 % of cases; however, persistent hypercalcemia was noted in up to 90 % of patients by 24 months [20, 21]. Finally, cinacalcet is well tolerated and appears to be effective in some case reports and small series [22–24], but long-term follow-up has been limited to a maximum of 60 months [22].

Our practice for MEN-1 patients with recurrent PHPT is to confirm the diagnosis with PTH, serum and urinary calcium levels, review the patient's list of medications, and begin with localization studies – most commonly a nuclear medicine parathyroid single-photon emission computed tomography (SPECT). In patients with suspected findings of one hyperfunctioning residual/ectopic gland, fine-needle aspiration (FNA) with PTH washout can be performed in hopes of planning for a limited cervical reexploration with simple resection of the offending gland. Reoperative intervention is tailored based on imaging and biopsy results. Discovery of multiple enlarged glands (Fig. 9.2) likely warrants bilateral neck reexploration. While reoperation is our preference, patients with a history of multiple or difficult *re*operations should be assessed for alternative strategies such as PetA or medical therapy. Although there is no optimal treatment, the final decision should be based on

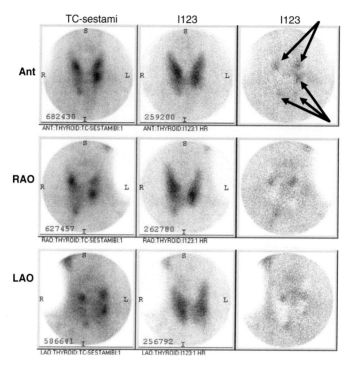

Fig. 9.2 SPECT revealing increased sestamibi uptake in a patient with potentially five hyperfunctioning glands

thoughtful and thorough discussions between experienced endocrine surgeons, endocrinologists, and the patient.

Outcome

In our patient we proceeded with a SPECT scan that identified a unilateral solitary mass, and ultrasound of the neck identified this to be 2 cm in size (Fig. 9.3a, b). Fine-needle aspiration with PTH

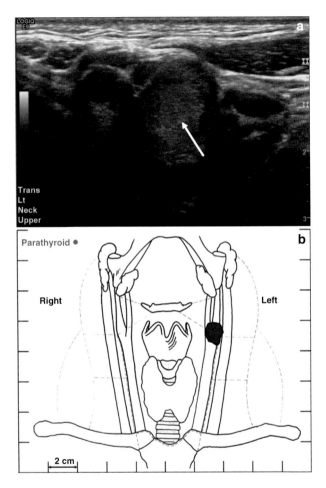

Fig. 9.3 (**a**) Ultrasound of the neck revealing a large mass (*arrow*) near the left carotid bifurcation. FNA biopsy of this lesion with PTH washout revealed parathyroid tissue with a PTH level of 1933 pg/mL. (**b**) Representative diagram of ultrasound shown in (a), highlighting the location of the mass in the neck

washout revealed parathyroid tissue with a PTH level of 1900 pg/mL. Reoperation was performed and the enlarged gland was removed with autotransplantation of a 40 mg portion to the left forearm. The patient's postoperative calcium and PTH normalized and she remains normocalcemic 2 years after surgery.

Clinical Pearls/Pitfalls
- Primary hyperparathyroidism (PHPT) in MEN-1 patients is due to asymmetric, multi-gland parathyroid adenomas.
- Initial surgery should begin with subtotal parathyroidectomy; ideally 3.5 glands are removed.
- Recurrent PHPT is expected long term and is common in most MEN-1 patients after the index parathyroidectomy; associated hypercalcemia may be difficult to treat.
- Recurrent PHPT after the initial subtotal parathyroidectomy should be thoroughly assessed by experienced endocrine surgeons and endocrinologists with a final treatment plan based on each individual patient. Surgical resection is optimal but offers no guarantee of long-term eucalcemia in MEN-1 patients.

Conflicts of Interest All authors state that they have no conflicts of interest.

References

1. Doherty GM. Multiple endocrine neoplasia type 1. J Surg Oncol. 2005;89:143–50.
2. Yip L, Ogilvie JB, Challinor SM, Salata RA, Thull DL, Yim JH, et al. Identification of multiple endocrine neoplasia type 1 in patients with apparent sporadic primary hyperparathyroidism. Surgery. 2008;144: 1002–6; discussion 1006–7.

 3. Schreinemakers JM, Pieterman CR, Scholten A, Vriens MR, Valk GD, Rinkes ID. The optimal surgical treatment for primary hyperparathyroidism in MEN1 patients: a systematic review. World J Surg. 2011;35:1993–2005.
 4. Thakker RV, Newey PJ, Walls GV, Bilezikian J, Dralle H, Ebeling PR, et al. Clinical practice guidelines for multiple endocrine neoplasia type 1 (MEN1). J Clin Endocrinol Metab. 2012;97:2990–3011.
 5. Doherty GM, Lairmore TC, DeBenedetti MK. Multiple endocrine neoplasia type 1 parathyroid adenoma development over time. World J Surg. 2004;28:1139–42.
 6. O'Riordain DS, O'Brien T, Grant CS, Weaver A, Gharib H, van Heerden JA. Surgical management of primary hyperparathyroidism in multiple endocrine neoplasia types 1 and 2. Surgery. 1993;114:1031–7; discussion 1037–9.
 7. Kivlen MH, Bartlett DL, Libutti SK, Skarulis MC, Marx SJ, Simonds WF, et al. Reoperation for hyperparathyroidism in multiple endocrine neoplasia type 1. Surgery. 2001;130:991–8.
 8. Brandi ML, Aurbach GD, Fitzpatrick LA, Quarto R, Spiegel AM, Bliziotes MM, et al. Parathyroid mitogenic activity in plasma from patients with familial multiple endocrine neoplasia type 1. N Engl J Med. 1986;314:1287–93.
 9. Zimering MB, Brandi ML, deGrange DA, Marx SJ, Streeten E, Katsumata N, et al. Circulating fibroblast growth factor-like substance in familial multiple endocrine neoplasia type 1. J Clin Endocrinol Metab. 1990;70:149–54.
10. Norton JA, Venzon DJ, Berna MJ, Alexander HR, Fraker DL, Libutti SK, et al. Prospective study of surgery for primary hyperparathyroidism (HPT) in multiple endocrine neoplasia-type 1 and Zollinger-Ellison syndrome: long-term outcome of a more virulent form of HPT. Ann Surg. 2008;247:501–10.
11. Arnalsteen LC, Alesina PF, Quiereux JL, Farrel SG, Patton FN, Carnaille BM, et al. Long-term results of less than total parathyroidectomy for hyperparathyroidism in multiple endocrine neoplasia type 1. Surgery. 2002;132:1119–24; discussion 1124–5.
12. Lambert LA, Shapiro SE, Lee JE, Perrier ND, Truong M, Wallace MJ, et al. Surgical treatment of hyperparathyroidism in patients with multiple endocrine neoplasia type 1. Arch Surg. 2005;140:374–82.
13. Tonelli F, Giudici F, Cavalli T, Brandi ML. Surgical approach in patients with hyperparathyroidism in multiple endocrine neoplasia type 1: total versus partial parathyroidectomy. Clinics. 2012;67 Suppl 1:155–60.

14. d'Alessandro AF, Montenegro FL, Brandao LG, Lourenco Jr DM, Toledo SA, Cordeiro AC. Supernumerary parathyroid glands in hyperparathyroidism associated with multiple endocrine neoplasia type 1. Rev Assoc Med Bras. 2012;58:323–7.
15. Lairmore TC, Govednik CM, Quinn CE, Sigmond BR, Lee CY, Jupiter DC. A randomized, prospective trial of operative treatments for hyperparathyroidism in patients with multiple endocrine neoplasia type 1. Surgery. 2014;156:1326–34; discussion 1334–5.
16. Waldmann J, Lopez CL, Langer P, Rothmund M, Bartsch DK. Surgery for multiple endocrine neoplasia type 1-associated primary hyperparathyroidism. Br J Surg. 2010;97:1528–34.
17. Elaraj DM, Skarulis MC, Libutti SK, Norton JA, Bartlett DL, Pingpank JF, et al. Results of initial operation for hyperparathyroidism in patients with multiple endocrine neoplasia type 1. Surgery. 2003;134:858–64; discussion 864–5.
18. Marx SJ. Etiologies of parathyroid gland dysfunction in primary hyperparathyroidism. J Bone Miner Res. 1991;6 Suppl 2:S19–24; discussion S31–2.
19. Hellman P, Skogseid B, Oberg K, Judlin C, Akerstrom G, Rastad J. Primary and reoperative parathyroid operations in hyperparathyroidism of multiple endocrine neoplasia type 1. Surgery. 1998;124:993–9.
20. Singh Ospina N, Thompson GB, Lee RA, Reading CC, Young Jr WF. Safety and efficacy of percutaneous parathyroid ethanol ablation in patients with recurrent primary hyperparathyroidism and multiple endocrine neoplasia type 1. J Clin Endocrinol Metab. 2015;100: E87–90.
21. Veldman MW, Reading CC, Farrell MA, Mullan BP, Wermers RA, Grant CS, et al. Percutaneous parathyroid ethanol ablation in patients with multiple endocrine neoplasia type 1. AJR Am J Roentgenol. 2008;191:1740–4.
22. Del Prete M, Marotta V, Ramundo V, Marciello F, Di Sarno A, Esposito R, et al. Impact of cinacalcet hydrochloride in clinical management of primary hyperparathyroidism in multiple endocrine neoplasia type 1. Minerva Endocrinol. 2013;38:389–94.
23. Falchetti A, Cilotti A, Vaggelli L, Masi L, Amedei A, Cioppi F, et al. A patient with MEN1-associated hyperparathyroidism, responsive to cinacalcet. Nat Clin Pract Endocrinol Metab. 2008;4:351–7.
24. Filopanti M, Verga U, Ermetici F, Olgiati L, Eller-Vainicher C, Corbetta S, et al. MEN1-related hyperparathyroidism: response to cinacalcet and its relationship with the calcium-sensing receptor gene variant Arg990Gly. Eur J Endocrinol. 2012;167:157–64.

Chapter 10
Parathyroid Carcinoma

Omair A. Shariq and Travis J. McKenzie

Case Study

A 71-year-old female presented to our clinic with a 3-month history of recurrent abdominal pain, nausea, and fatigue. She had a history of coronary artery disease, hypertension, and osteoarthritis. She denied significant alcohol use and was a non-smoker. She also denied any therapeutic radiation exposure or family history of cancer. On clinical examination, she appeared dehydrated and lethargic but was hemodynamically stable. A right-sided firm, irregular, non-tender mass was palpable in the area of the right thyroid lobe measuring approximately 3 cm by examination.

O.A. Shariq, MRCS
Department of Surgery, Mayo Clinic, Rochester, MN, USA
e-mail: shariq.omair@mayo.edu

T.J. McKenzie, MD (✉)
Department of Surgery, Mayo College of Medicine, Mayo Clinic, Rochester, MN, USA
e-mail: mckenzie.travis@mayo.edu

A.E. Kearns, R.A. Wermers (eds.), *Hyperparathyroidism: A Clinical Casebook*, DOI 10.1007/978-3-319-25880-5_10,
© Mayo Foundation for Medical Education and Research 2016

Laboratory investigations showed raised levels of total serum calcium 14.0 mg/dL (nl. 8.9–10.1), phosphorus 2.2 mg/dL (nl. 2.5–4.5), and parathyroid hormone (PTH) 239 pg/mL (nl. 10–65). Cervical ultrasonography (Fig. 10.1) revealed a 3.5-cm heterogeneous, hypervascular lobulated mass with calcification along the posterior aspect of the right lower thyroid lobe. There was no concerning cervical lymphadenopathy. Tc-99 m sestamibi single-photon emission computed tomography (SPECT-CT) showed a large focus of heterogeneous sestamibi uptake in a region corresponding with the mass identified on cervical ultrasound.

Diagnosis and Assessment

Our patient's clinical presentation is consistent with hypercalcemia due to primary hyperparathyroidism. Parathyroid carcinoma (PC) is a rare endocrine malignancy, accounting for around 1 % of cases of primary hyperparathyroidism [1]. This infrequent, but potentially life-threatening, clinical entity was first reported by Wilder of Mayo Clinic in 1929 [2]. Conditions that appear to result in an increased risk of PC include multiple endocrine neoplasia type 1 [3], autosomal dominant familial isolated hyperparathyroidism [4], and hyperparathyroidism-jaw tumor syndrome due to mutation of the CDC73 gene [5].

PC presents a diagnostic and therapeutic challenge due to overlapping features with benign primary hyperparathyroidism and the lack of specific differentiating characteristics for malignancy. However, patients with PC typically have a serum PTH greater than five times the upper limit of normal and calcium levels in excess of 14 mg/dL, significantly higher than those with parathyroid adenoma or hyperplasia [6]. Unlike parathyroid adenoma, which has a female preponderance, PC affects both sexes equally, with an earlier median age of diagnosis in the fifth decade [7]. The findings of a palpable neck mass and

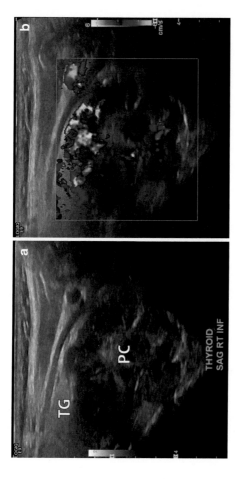

Fig. 10.1 Sonogram of the right side of the neck, sagittal view. (**a**) A mass (*PC*) measuring approximately 3.5 × 2.6 × 2.9 cm is seen lying along the inferior and posterior aspect of the right lobe of the thyroid gland (*TG*). It is heterogeneous with lobulated margins and has internal calcifications. Both lobes of the thyroid are normal in size with normal vascularity. (**b**) The mass is hypervascular on color Doppler flow imaging

dysphonia related to recurrent laryngeal nerve palsy as well as the combination of severe renal and bone disease are also suggestive of malignancy [7, 8].

The diagnosis of PC relies on a high index of suspicion, taking into account the patient's clinical presentation, laboratory studies, imaging, and histopathology. The vast majority of PCs are functioning neoplasms, with clinical features and symptoms resulting from excessive secretion of PTH rather than local infiltration or mass effect from the neoplasm itself. Initial laboratory evaluation should include measurement of total serum calcium, PTH, and serum creatinine and an assessment of overall fluid and electrolyte status.

Ultrasound and sestamibi scintigraphy provide information on localization and the extent of the neoplasm, though neither is specific for carcinoma. Nonetheless, evidence of tumor invasion, irregular margins, and cervical node enlargement on ultrasound may raise suspicion for PC [9]. SPECT-CT with sestamibi, as utilized in this case, provides three-dimensional information with improved sensitivity for the detection of hyperfunctioning parathyroid glands [10]. Computerized tomography and magnetic resonance imaging, although not typically utilized on initial evaluation, may be useful adjuncts to ultrasonography in assessing for distant metastases in the chest or abdomen. Selective venous catheterization and PTH measurement may also be useful if noninvasive tests are equivocal or negative.

Fine needle aspiration (FNA) is not recommended in the setting of suspected PC due to the inability of cytology to differentiate between benign and malignant disease and the potential risk of ectopic tumor seeding [11].

Management

Prior to operative intervention, patients may require urgent management of dehydration, hypercalcemia, and associated metabolic abnormalities. Our patient was admitted for aggressive hydration with saline, initiation of a loop diuretic to promote calcium excretion, and administration of pamidronate. Following this, the decision was made to proceed to the operating room.

The gold standard treatment for PC is en bloc surgical resection [8]. Removal of any contiguous tissues to which the neoplasm adheres is necessary to achieve complete resection. This frequently includes the ipsilateral thyroid lobe and may necessitate resection of the ipsilateral recurrent laryngeal nerve. Ipsilateral compartment VI central neck dissection with removal of all lymphatic tissue should be performed. Care must be taken to avoid rupturing the capsule of the neoplasm, as this increases the likelihood of malignant parathyromatosis [12]. As highest chance of cure is obtainable if en bloc resection is carried out at the initial operation, a high index of suspicion for PC is therefore paramount. Chemotherapy and radiation have generally shown disappointing results [13].

Histopathological diagnosis is challenging, and while early pathologic criteria suggested the presence of a trabecular growth pattern, capsular invasion, vascular invasion, dense fibrous bands, and mitotic figures as suggestive of malignancy [14], later studies have shown that none of these are pathognomonic and may exist in parathyroid adenomas [15, 16]. Thus, the only unequivocal proof of malignancy is the local invasion of contiguous structures noted during surgery or the presence of distant metastasis.

In the postoperative period, serum calcium levels should be closely monitored. Adequate replacement with oral calcium, calcitriol, and intravenous calcium gluconate may be necessary to avoid symptomatic hypocalcemia associated with the "hungry bone syndrome." When intravenous calcium supplementation is necessary, we recommend utilizing a central venous route as peripheral venous calcium supplementation can rarely result in local tissue necrosis [17].

Recurrence occurs in more than 50 % of cases [8, 18], most commonly in the neck, followed by the lungs, liver, and bone

[19]. The majority of patients benefit from debulking of recurrent disease, if technically feasible, as palliation from the effects of hypercalcemia and hyperparathyroidism. Unfortunately, reoperation is rarely curative and eventual relapse is likely.

Outcome

Intraoperatively, a 3.5-cm heterogeneous, firm mass was found posterior to the right thyroid lobe with invasion into the thyroid parenchyma and involving the right recurrent laryngeal nerve. En bloc resection of the right parathyroid carcinoma with right thyroid lobectomy, right recurrent laryngeal nerve excision, and ipsilateral central lymph node dissection was therefore performed. Intraoperative PTH dropped from a baseline of 193–17.4 pg/mL 15 min after removal. The patient was discharged the following day without evidence of hypocalcemia. At 6-month follow-up, serum calcium and parathyroid hormone were within normal limits, and cervical ultrasound demonstrated no evidence of recurrent or persistent structural disease.

Clinical Pearls/Pitfalls
- PC is a rare cause of hyperparathyroidism.
- Overlapping features with benign hyperparathyroidism can make the diagnosis challenging.
- Compared with benign primary hyperparathyroidism, patients with PC are more likely to present with symptoms, a neck mass, bone and renal disease, marked hypercalcemia, and very high serum PTH levels.

- Ultrasound, sestamibi, and SPECT-CT are helpful in localizing and identifying the extent of the tumor. FNA should be avoided.
- A definitive diagnosis of PC can only be made if the tumor is noted to be invading into surrounding tissues or distant metastases are found.
- Patients have the highest chance of cure if en bloc resection is carried out at the initial operation. Thus, preoperative suspicion and intraoperative recognition of PC are essential.
- Correction of hypercalcemia and dehydration preoperatively is essential in preventing possible renal failure and cardiac arrest.

Conflicts of Interest All authors state that they have no conflicts of interest.

References

1. Givi B, Shah JP. Parathyroid carcinoma. Clin Oncol (R Coll Radiol). 2010;22(6):498–507.
2. Wilder RM. Hyperparathyroidism: tumor of the parathyroid glands associated with osteitis fibrosa. Endocrinology. 1929;13:231–44.
3. Wassif WS, Moniz CF, Friedman E, et al. Familial isolated hyperparathyroidism: a distinct genetic entity with an increased risk of parathyroid cancer. J Clin Endocrinol Metab. 1993;77:1485–9.
4. Agha A, Carpenter R, Bhattacharya S, Edmonson SJ, Carlsen E, Monson JP. Parathyroid carcinoma in multiple endocrine neoplasia type 1 (MEN1) syndrome: two case reports of an unrecognised entity. J Endocrinol Invest. 2007;30:145e149.
5. Sharretts JM, Simonds WF. Clinical and molecular genetics of parathyroid neoplasms. Best Pract Res Clin Endocrinol Metab. 2010;24(3): 491–502.

6. Robert JH, Trombetti A, Garcia A, Pache JC, Herrmann F, Spiliopoulos A, Rizzoli R. Primary hyperparathyroidism: can parathyroid carcinoma be anticipated on clinical and biochemical grounds? Report of nine cases and review of the literature. Ann Surg Oncol. 2005;12(7):526.

7. Wynne AG, van Heerden J, Carney JA, Fitzpatrick LA. Parathyroid carcinoma: clinical and pathologic features in 43 patients. Medicine (Baltimore). 1992;71(4):197–205.

8. Shane E. Clinical review 122: parathyroid carcinoma. J Clin Endocrinol Metab. 2001;86:485e493.

9. Johnston LB, Carroll MJ, Britton KE, Lowe DG, Shand W, Besser GM, et al. The accuracy of parathyroid gland localization in primary hyperparathyroidism using Sestamibi radionuclide imaging. J Clin Endocrinol Metab. 1996;81:346.

10. Chen CC, Holder LE, Scovili WA, Tehan AM, Gann DS. Comparison of parathyroid imaging with technetium-99m-pertechnetate/sestamibi subtraction, double-phase technetium-99m-sestamibi and technetium-99m-sestamibi SPECT. J Nucl Med. 1997;38(6):834–9.

11. Spinelli C, Bonadio AG, Berti P, Materazzi G, Miccoli P. Cutaneous spreading of parathyroid carcinoma after fine needle aspiration cytology. J Endocrinol Invest. 2000;23:255e257.

12. Koea JB, Shaw JH. Parathyroid cancer: biology and management. Surg Oncol. 1999;8:155e165.

13. Obara T, Fujimoto Y. Diagnosis and treatment of patients with parathyroid carcinoma: an update and review. World J Surg. 1991;15(6):738.

14. Schantz A, Castleman B. Parathyroid carcinoma. A study of 70 cases. Cancer. 1973;31:600e605.

15. McKeown PP, McGarity WC, Sewell CW. Carcinoma of the parathyroid gland: is it overdiagnosed? A report of three cases. Am J Surg. 1984;147:292e298.

16. Bondeson L, Sandelin K, Grimelius L. Histopathological variables and DNA cytometry in parathyroid carcinoma. Am J Surg Pathol. 1993;17(8):820–9.

17. Klein R. Hypocalcemia. In: Loriaux L, editor. Endocrine emergencies: recognition and treatment. New York: Springer; 2010. p. 149–60.

18. Kebebew E. Parathyroid carcinoma. Curr Treat Options Oncol. 2001;2:347e354.

19. Kebebew E, Arici C, Duh QY, Clark OH. Localization and reoperation results for persistent and recurrent parathyroid carcinoma. Arch Surg. 2001;136(8):878–85.

Chapter 11
Primary Hyperparathyroidism Due to Parathyromatosis

Melanie L. Richards

Case Presentation

A 61-year-old woman was referred for recurrent primary hyperparathyroidism (PHPT). She reported symptoms of fatigue, joint discomfort, and memory problems. A serum calcium level was 12.8 mg/dl (normal, 8.9–10.1 mg/dl), and a parathyroid hormone level (PTH) was 224 pg/ml (normal, 15–65 pg/ml). Her 24-h urine calcium was 444 mg. A bone mineral density study was unremarkable. There was a remote history of nephrolithiasis, and a recent abdominal film was negative for nephrolithiasis. She initially presented with hypercalcemia (serum calcium 11.0 mg/dl) at age 41 and was diagnosed with PHPT. At that time observation was recommended. Her past medical history was significant for childhood radiation therapy for ear infections. Family history was significant for a maternal aunt with PHPT.

At age 50 she developed nephrolithiasis and her calcium had increased to 13.1 mg/dl. Surgery was recommended, and the

M.L. Richards, MD, MHPE
Department of Surgery, Mayo College of Medicine, Mayo Clinic,
Rochester, MN, USA
e-mail: richards.melanie@mayo.edu

A.E. Kearns, R.A. Wermers (eds.), *Hyperparathyroidism:
A Clinical Casebook*, DOI 10.1007/978-3-319-25880-5_11,
© Mayo Foundation for Medical Education and Research 2016

patient underwent resection of a 3-cm right superior parathyroid gland at an outside institution. A right thyroid lobectomy was also performed because of nodular thyroid disease and history of radiation exposure. No exploration of the left neck was performed. The pathology report stated that she had a parathyroid carcinoma. Her calcium normalized and remained normal until 4 years postoperatively when she had a minimal elevation of the ionized calcium and a PTH of 109 pg/ml. Her pathology slides were rereviewed and reported as an atypical parathyroid adenoma. Parathyroid sestamibi imaging showed uptake in the region of the left superior thyroid. No intervention was recommended at that time.

Assessment and Diagnosis

Surgery in PHPT is successful 97 % of the time, and most operative failures are related to persistent PHPT [1]. Recurrent PHPT is diagnosed when a patient develops hypercalcemia after a period of at least 6 months of normocalcemia following parathyroidectomy [2]. Patients that have persistent or recurrent PHPT following removal of a hypercellular parathyroid gland/s most likely have multiglandular disease, with hyperplasia being more common than double adenomas. Parathyroid carcinoma is responsible for fewer than 5 % of operative failures [3]. However, approximately 50 % of patients with parathyroid carcinoma will have a recurrence. Parathyromatosis is the rarest cause of persistent or recurrent PHPT.

Parathyromatosis was first described in 1975 and has been limited to case reports in the medical literature [4]. Patients with parathyromatosis have sites (usually multiple) of hyperfunctioning parathyroid tissue that has implanted within soft tissues of the neck and occasionally the mediastinum. The most likely cause of parathyromatosis is disruption of a benign hypercellular parathyroid gland at the time of the initial operation. Patients at risk for parathyroid disruption are those with larger parathyroid glands. Parathyroid carcinomas are also typically larger and may lead to parathyromatosis. It is controversial whether parathyromatosis in parathyroid cancer develops from tumor disruption and seeding or whether it is a locoregional spread of the cancer. Those with secondary hyperparathyroidism (HPT) who undergo subtotal or total parathyroidectomy have been reported to have the highest risk of developing parathyromatosis [3]. Patients that have mediastinal parathyromatosis will typically have it intrathymic, and it is often attributed to multiple parathyroid embryologic rests becoming hyperplastic, either from secondary HPT or with familial PHPT [5]. These embryologic rests can also be located adjacent to the thyroid and in the perithyroidal fat [6].

This patient presents a unique challenge because she has risk factors for multiglandular disease, as well as for parathyromatosis and possible parathyroid carcinoma. Having recurrence alone suggests multiglandular disease, and in this patient it could be either familial PHPT or related to a history of external radiation therapy. A prolonged period of normocalcemia and the absence of a critically high calcium level support the diagnosis of an atypical parathyroid adenoma rather than a parathyroid carcinoma. The histopathology of parathyroid carcinoma typically will show capsular, vascular, or lymph node invasion in conjunction with a trabecular growth pattern and increased mitoses (>1/10 high-power fields) [7]. It has been found that there is not a single molecular marker for parathyroid cancer but that a molecular profile consisting of loss of parafibromin and Rb expression and an overexpression of galectin-3 supports the diagnosis of parathyroid cancer [8]. Parathyromatosis does not appear to be a low-grade parathyroid carcinoma. Having her pathology rereviewed with current histopathologic techniques and molecular studies was helpful to confirm a diagnosis of an atypical parathyroid adenoma, as opposed to the initial diagnosis of parathyroid cancer.

The parathyroid gland removed at the primary operation was reported to measure 3 cm in size, which would be classified as very large and also at risk for parathyromatosis. Parathyroid imaging that localizes can be utilized to differentiate between the causes of recurrent PHPT. It may localize hypercellular parathyroid glands in the anatomic region of a normal parathyroid gland or an ectopic location consistent with embryologic development of a parathyroid gland (e.g., carotid sheath, thymus, piriform sinus, intrathyroidal). Localization in the soft tissue, typically in multiple areas, indicates parathyromatosis. Neck ultrasound is more helpful for localization than sestamibi parathyroid imaging secondary to the small size of the implants and the more superficial location in the subcutaneous fat and strap muscles.

The decision to proceed with localization is based on whether the patient is a surgical candidate. The success of a reoperation is increased when concordant findings are found on two or more imaging modalities [9]. We have reported curative reoperation in 89 % of all patients with persistent or recurrent PHPT [10]. Patients with parathyromatosis are difficult to cure secondary to the multiple sites of implanted tissue in the reoperative field. A comprehensive literature review of 35 patients with parathyromatosis (both PHPT and secondary HPT) reported 25/35 (71 %) cases with documented persistent or recurrent disease [3].

Management

The patient underwent parathyroid subtraction imaging with single-photon emission computed tomography (SPECT) views. The images showed uptake in area of the right thyroid bed, which are shown to be more anterior in the pretracheal area on SPECT (Figs. 11.1 and 11.2). A neck ultrasound showed multiple nodules in the neck (Fig. 11.3). There were a 9-mm nodule in the right thyroid bed and a 1.3-cm nodule inferior to the left lobe of the thyroid, both corresponding to the abnormalities seen on the

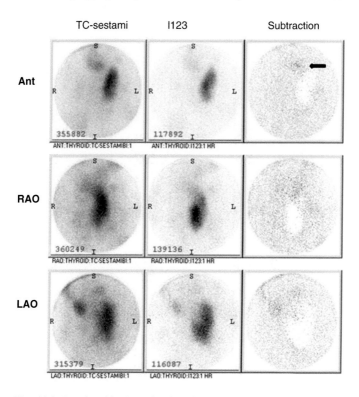

Fig. 11.1 Parathyroid subtraction imaging showing uptake in the pretracheal region

parathyroid scan. There were three nodules within the left thyroid gland (the right lobe was surgically absent) with the largest measuring 1.8 cm. There were two nodules felt to be enlarged lymph nodes located pretracheal within the subcutaneous tissue, the measuring 1.2 cm and 0.7 cm. There was also a small superficial "lymph node" superficial to the left lobe of the thyroid gland measuring 5 mm. The largest thyroid nodule and one of the large lymph nodes underwent fine needle aspiration biopsy. The thyroid nodule biopsy was nondiagnostic, and the pretracheal

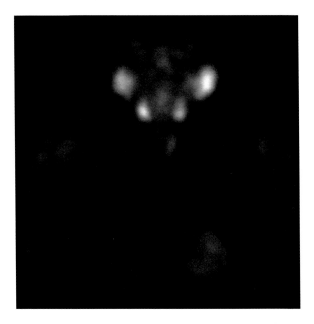

Fig. 11.2 SPECT sestamibi parathyroid imaging showing multiple pretracheal nodules

nodule was neoplastic with a reported differential of parathyroid versus follicular versus medullary. A vocal cord assessment was normal. Neck exploration was recommended for removal of the multiple implants and a completion thyroidectomy because of the nondiagnostic biopsy and history of external radiation.

She underwent cervical exploration with intraoperative PTH monitoring and intraoperative laryngeal nerve monitoring. Completion thyroidectomy confirmed multiple adenomatous nodules. The left inferior parathyroid gland was enlarged and excised, confirmed to be hypercellular and weighing 200 mg. The left superior parathyroid gland was grossly normal in size, and a biopsy confirmed parathyroid tissue. Adjacent to his was a small implant of hypercellular parathyroid tissue. There were six subcutaneous

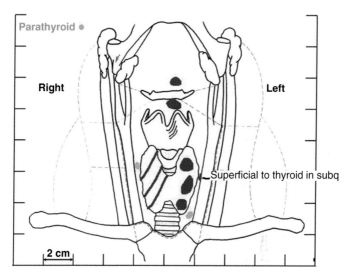

Fig. 11.3 Neck ultrasound demonstrating multiple subcutaneous nodules ranging in size from 0.5 to 1.2 cm, multiple nodules in the left thyroid (largest 1.8 cm), 9-mm nodule in the right thyroid bed, and a 1.3-cm nodule inferior to the left thyroid

and intramuscular implants of hypercellular parathyroid tissue, several with atypia, excised. They ranged in size from 40 to 920 mg. A total of 1,540 mg of hypercellular parathyroid tissue was excised. Methylation-inhibited binding protein-1 (MIB-1) stain showed a moderate proliferative rate consistent with parathyromatosis. Intraoperative PTH levels normalized to 26 pg/ml.

Outcome

She remained normocalcemic for 8 months after her cervical re-exploration. At that time she had a mildly elevated calcium of

10.3 mg/dl. She was asymptomatic and followed conservatively for two more years. She developed progressive hypercalcemia and became symptomatic. At that time she underwent re-exploration at an outside institution with removal of three subcutaneous implants.

Clinical Pearls/Pitfalls
- Care should be taken to minimize disruption of hyper-cellular parathyroid glands at the initial operation. If there is disruption of the parathyroid gland, then it is critical to remove any identifiable fragments of parathyroid tissue.
- Parathyromatosis should be considered in the differential for patients with persistent or recurrent PHPT, particularly if they had a history of a large hypercellular parathyroid gland.
- Multimodality imaging can be helpful for creating an intraoperative road map to identify the multiple sites of parathyromatosis.
- Intraoperative PTH monitoring is a useful adjunct that may reduce the incidence of persistent PHPT.
- Parathyromatosis may be difficult to cure in a single reoperation. It is important to have long-term follow-up to identify persistent and recurrent disease.

Conflicts of Interest All authors state that they have no conflicts of interest.

References

1. Richards ML, Thompson GB, Farley DR, Grant CS. An optimal algorithm for intraoperative parathyroid hormone monitoring. Arch Surg. 2011;146(3):280–5.

2. Wells Jr SA, Debenedetti MK, Doherty GM. Recurrent or persistent hyperparathyroidism. J Bone Miner Res. 2002;17 Suppl 2:N158–N16.
3. Hage MP, Salti I, El-Hajj Fuleihan G. Parathyromatosis: a rare yet problematic etiology of recurrent and persistent hyperparathyroidism. Metabolism. 2012;61(6):762–75.
4. Palmer JA, Brown WA, Kerr WH, Rosen IB, Watters NA. The surgical aspects of hyperparathyroidism. Arch Surg. 1975;110:1004–7.
5. Reddick RL, Costa JC, Marx SJ. Parathyroid hyperplasia and parathyromatosis. Lancet. 1977;1:549.
6. Aly A, Douglas M. Embryonic parathyroid rests occur commonly and have implications in the management of secondary hyperparathyroidism. ANZ J Surg. 2003;73:284–8.
7. Schantz A, Castleman B. Parathyroid carcinoma. A study of 70 cases. Cancer. 1973;31:600–5.
8. Fernandez-Ranvier GG, Khanafshar E, Tacha D, Wong M, Kebebew E, Duh QY, Clark OH. Defining a molecular phenotype for benign and malignant parathyroid tumors. Cancer. 2009;115:334–44.
9. Thompson GB, Grant CS, Perrier ND, Harman R, Hodgson SF, Ilstrup D, van Heerden JA. Reoperative parathyroid surgery in the era of sestamibi scanning and intraoperative parathyroid hormone monitoring. Arch Surg. 1999;134(7):699–704; discussion 704–5.
10. Richards ML, Thompson GB, Farley DR, Grant CS. Reoperative parathyroidectomy in 228 patients during the era of minimal-access surgery and intraoperative parathyroid hormone monitoring. Am J Surg. 2008;196(6):937–42; discussion 942–3.

Chapter 12
Familial Hypocalciuric Hypercalcemia

Ann E. Kearns and Robert A. Wermers

Case Presentation

A 38-year-old woman is referred for evaluation of persistent primary hyperparathyroidism (PHPT). Two years prior, hypercalcemia was detected during evaluation of "hurting all over." A diagnosis of PHPT was made based on calcium 11.6 mg/dL and PTH 62 pg/mL. A parathyroid scan was reported not to localize a potential parathyroid adenoma. She underwent a neck exploration. Pathology revealed that only one of the six tissue samples contained parathyroid tissue and that parathyroid tissue appeared normal. Hypercalcemia persisted postoperatively (11.8 mg/dL) with a normal PTH (46 pg/mL). A second parathyroid scan was again negative. She reports that her father had hypercalcemia,

A.E. Kearns, MD, PhD (✉) • R.A. Wermers, MD
Division of Endocrinology, Diabetes, Metabolism, and Nutrition,
Department of Internal Medicine, Mayo College of Medicine,
Mayo Clinic, Rochester, MN, USA
e-mail: kearns.ann@mayo.edu; wermers.robert@mayo.edu

A.E. Kearns, R.A. Wermers (eds.), *Hyperparathyroidism:*
A Clinical Casebook, DOI 10.1007/978-3-319-25880-5_12,
© Mayo Foundation for Medical Education and Research 2016

but no other details or a specific diagnosis was known. She had no history of head and neck irradiation or lithium therapy, and no history of kidney stones. Current medications did not include thiazide-type diuretics or calcium supplements. Physical examination was normal, with note of a well-healed neck scar.

Her current laboratory evaluation revealed calcium 11.0 mg/dL (8.9–10.2 mg/dL), PTH 63 pg/mL (15–65 pg/mL), 24 h urine calcium 40 mg/24 h, and calculated calcium/creatinine clearance ratio 0.004. Imaging of the kidneys was negative for kidney stones and bone density was normal in the hip, spine, and radius.

Assessment and Diagnosis

The initial approach to a patient with persistent hypercalcemia after parathyroidectomy includes a review of the original diagnosis of PHPT and a review of the operative report and pathology report from the initial surgery. Diagnostic considerations include the possibility of an ectopic parathyroid adenoma or inadequate neck exploration, parathyroid carcinoma, and multigland parathyroid disease (Table 12.1). In this case the history of hypercalcemia in the patient's father suggests possible familial disorders of PHPT which include familial hypocalciuric hypercalcemia (FHH), multiple endocrine neoplasia (MEN) syndromes, hyperparathyroidism-jaw tumor, familial isolated hyperparathyroidism, and non-syndromic PHPT [1]. There are now three MEN syndromes but PHPT is most commonly seen in MEN type 1 which has common manifestations of pancreatic and pituitary tumors also. Hyperparathyroidism-jaw tumor syndrome is characterized by parathyroid tumors including carcinoma and fibro-osseous jaw tumors. In all the familial disorders except FHH, the urinary calcium is usually elevated as in sporadic PHPT.

Table 12.1 Diagnostic considerations in confirmed albumin-corrected hypercalcemia with inappropriately normal or elevated parathyroid hormone level

Sporadic primary hyperparathyroidism	Familial primary hyperparathyroidism
Adenoma (85 %)	Isolated
Hyperplasia (15 %)	MEN1
Carcinoma (<1 %)	MEN2A
	MEN4
	Hyperparathyroidism-jaw tumor
Familial hypocalciuric hypercalcemia	Tertiary hyperparathyroidism
Autoimmune hypocalciuric hypercalcemia	Chronic renal failure
Lithium-associated hypercalcemia	Thiazide-associated hypercalcemia

FHH is an autosomal dominant disorder with a nearly 100 % penetrance of hypercalcemia at all ages most commonly caused by a heterozygous inactivating mutation of the *CASR* gene, which encodes the calcium-sensing receptor (CaSR) [2, 3]. Homozygous inactivating mutations are found in neonatal severe hyperparathyroidism. The CaSR is a critical part of calcium homeostasis through its role in regulating PTH secretion and renal tubular reabsorption of calcium. The result of the inactivating mutation is an increase in the set point for calcium-induced suppression of PTH secretion and renal tubular calcium reabsorption. The CaSR is a typical G-protein-coupled receptor that is widely expressed both in tissues with direct involvement with calcium homeostasis such as the parathyroid glands and the kidneys but also in tissues without a role in calcium homeostasis [4].

Initially FHH was thought to be only caused by mutations in the *CASR* gene (FHH1 in ≈65 %). However, additional loss of function mutations has been identified in the G-alpha subunit 11 (*GNA11* gene) (FHH2 in ≈15 %) [5] and the adaptor-related protein complex, sigma 1 subunit (*AP2S1* gene) (FHH3 in ≈ 20 %), which encodes the adapter-protein 2 sigma subunit [6]. These mutations interfere with the normal signaling of the CaSR complex. On a clinical basis, these are indistinguishable from FHH caused by inactivation of the CaSR.

Distinguishing PHPT and FHH can be challenging, especially in the absence of a family history. Clear evidence of prior normal calcium values over time would argue against FHH and for PHPT. Individuals with FHH do not present with the classic complications seen in PHPT such as nephrolithiasis. However, serum PTH levels are elevated in 5–25 % of FHH subjects [7], and although renal calcium to creatinine clearance ratio below 0.01 is highly suggestive of FHH, there is considerable overlap in this ratio between FHH and PHPT. The risk of osteoporosis in individuals with FHH is similar to that expected in the general population, and forearm bone mineral density (frequently low in PHPT) was not found to be a reliable diagnostic tool to discriminate the two disorders [8].

Management

The findings of a low calcium/creatinine clearance ratio and a father with hypercalcemia were suggestive of FHH. The patient agreed to genetic testing of the *CASR* gene for mutations that cause inactivation and would suggest a diagnosis of FHH. The following heterozygous sequence change was detected: Exon, 7; DNA change, c.2243C>G; and amino acid change, p. P748R. This alteration is known to be disease associated with FHH. The inactivating mutations in the *CASR* gene giving rise to FHH now number over 150 and can occur anywhere in the coding region but most frequently are reported in the N-terminal extracellular domain and the signal transduction domain [4]. Variable elevations in serum calcium levels are seen with different *CASR* gene mutations. *CASR* gene testing can be falsely negative in approximately 30 % if the mutation is outside of the tested coding exons. Autoantibodies to the CaSR (autoimmune hypocalciuric hypercalcemia) have been reported to result in a similar syndrome of hypocalciuric hypercalcemia [9].

Outcome

The patient was reassured that this finding did not require additional surgery. She received counseling about the autosomal dominant mode of inheritance and was advised to inform family members who may have inherited this disorder.

Clinical Pearls
- Persistent PHPT after an initial neck exploration requires reassessment of the underlying diagnosis.
- Several disorders can produce familial PHPT, but FHH is classically associated with low urinary calcium and the others are not.
- There is some overlap in the biochemical parameters reported in PHPT and FHH.
- Genetic testing should be considered in suspected cases of FHH because documenting a disease-associated mutation can eliminate unnecessary surgery.

Conflict of Interest All authors state that they have no conflicts of interest.

References

1. Thakker RV, Familial and hereditary forms of primary hyperparathyroidism. In: Bilezikian JP, editor. The parathyroids. Elsevier; 2015. p. 341–88.

2. Law Jr WM, Heath 3rd H. Familial benign hypercalcemia (hypo-calciuric hypercalcemia). Clinical and pathogenetic studies in 21 families. Ann Intern Med. 1985;102(4):511–9.
3. Marx SJ, et al. The hypocalciuric or benign variant of familial hypercalcemia: clinical and biochemical features in fifteen kindreds. Medicine. 1981;60(6):397–412.
4. Ward BK, et al. The role of the calcium-sensing receptor in human disease. Clin Biochem. 2012;45(12):943–53.
5. Nesbit MA, et al. Mutations affecting G-protein subunit alpha11 in hypercalcemia and hypocalcemia. N Engl J Med. 2013; 368(26):2476–86.
6. Nesbit MA, et al. Mutations in AP2S1 cause familial hypocalciuric hypercalcemia type 3. Nat Genet. 2013;45(1):93–7.
7. Christensen SE, et al. Familial hypocalciuric hypercalcaemia: a review. Curr Opin Endocrinol Diabetes Obes. 2011;18(6):359–70.
8. Isaksen T, et al. Forearm bone mineral density in familial hypocalciuric hypercalcemia and primary hyperparathyroidism: a comparative study. Calcif Tissue Int. 2011;89(4):285–94.
9. Kifor O, et al. A syndrome of hypocalciuric hypercalcemia caused by autoantibodies directed at the calcium-sensing receptor. J Clin Endocrinol Metab. 2003;88(1):60–72.

Chapter 13
Medical Management of Primary Hyperparathyroidism

Ann E. Kearns

Case Presentation

A 53-year-old woman is seen for persistent primary hyperpara-thyroidism (PHPT). She has a complex past history of PHPT. She was originally found to be hypercalcemic at age 39 on routine blood tests performed prior to initiating medication for psoria-sis. Testing confirmed the presence of PHPT: calcium 14.1 mg/dL (8.9–10.2 mg/dL), parathyroid hormone (PTH) 30 pg/mL (1.0–5.2 pg/mL), and 24 h urine calcium 321 mg/24 h. She had no family history of hypercalcemia or endocrine tumors. She had no personal history of kidney stones, head and neck irradia-tion, lithium use, or fractures. She underwent her first neck exploration with removal of a right inferior parathyroid ade-noma weighing 1.56 g. Her calcium never completely normal-ized. She subsequently has undergone a total of five neck

A.E. Kearns, MD, PhD
Division of Endocrinology, Diabetes, Metabolism, and Nutrition,
Department of Internal Medicine, Mayo College of Medicine,
Mayo Clinic, Rochester, MN, USA
e-mail: kearns.ann@mayo.edu

A.E. Kearns, R.A. Wermers (eds.), *Hyperparathyroidism:*
A Clinical Casebook, DOI 10.1007/978-3-319-25880-5_13,
© Mayo Foundation for Medical Education and Research 2016

explorations without complete resolution of hypercalcemia. Her bone density is normal in the lumbar spine and hips and osteopenic at the one-third radius with a T-score of −1.6. She has no recurrent laryngeal nerve damage. Her current laboratories show calcium 11.9 mg/dL (8.9−10.2 mg/dL) and PTH 215 pg/mL (10−65 pg/mL). She has symptoms of fatigue and depression. Her only other medical problem is psoriasis. Parathyroid scan, neck ultrasound, and a four-dimensional computed tomography (4D CT) scan do not identify abnormal parathyroid gland.

Assessment and Diagnosis

Surgery is the treatment of choice for PHPT and is highly curative of the disorder. However, in the reoperative case for persistent (as this patient has) or recurrent PHPT, the cure rate is dramatically reduced with increasing number of operations [1]. Medical management of patients with PHPT is considered when surgery is not recommended due to comorbid medical conditions, unsuccessful or complicated prior surgery, or based on patient choice. Patients not undergoing surgery should be assessed for current complications of PHPT with appropriate imaging (e.g., bone density testing, kidney imaging for nephrolithiasis) and blood tests to assess calcium and kidney function.

A recent consensus statement on medical management of PHPT recommended that patients with PHPT be advised to consume the same amount of calcium as the general population and vitamin D intake should be adequate to maintain levels at least greater than 20 ng/mL [2]. Repletion of vitamin D deficiency in PHPT has been shown to lower bone turnover [3]. Therapy with oral bisphosphonates (alendronate and risedronate), estrogen, or raloxifene has been shown to have beneficial effects on bone density and bone turnover in PHPT [2]. No long-term trials have been performed with fracture outcomes. In one study, surgery was more beneficial to bone density than risedronate [4]. No consistent effects have been seen on serum calcium with use of oral bisphosphonates or raloxifene in PHPT. Therefore, it seems reasonable to use bisphosphonates, especially alendronate which is the best studied in PHPT, to attenuate the effects of PHPT on bone density in patients with osteoporosis or high fracture risk. The duration of bisphosphonate therapy use in PHPT has not been studied and may be determined by periodic assessment of fracture risk and bone density. A drug holiday may be appropriate as in general postmenopausal osteoporosis.

Cinacalcet is a calcimimetic drug that increases the sensitivity of the calcium-sensing receptor on the parathyroid glands, thereby reducing PTH secretion and serum calcium. In a recent short-term double-blind randomized placebo-controlled trial, cinacalcet normalized calcium in 76 % of PHPT subjects and PTH was reduced [5]. A pooled analysis similarly demonstrated that cinacalcet was effective in lowering calcium across a spectrum of PHPT including failed parathyroidectomy [6]. However, cinacalcet did not have demonstrable benefits on bone density. A small prospective study suggests that cinacalcet with appropriate diet may lower the rate of formation of kidney stones in PHPT [7]. Symptom improvement in PHPT treated with cinacalcet has not been extensively studied but a small study of 17 patients reported improvement in Medical Outcomes Study (MOS) Short Form 36 (SF-36) scores with cinacalcet treatment [8]. As with bisphosphonate use in PHPT, the potential long duration of use of cinacalcet in this setting is unstudied. The high incidence of side effects including nausea, vomiting, and diarrhea may limit use. Hypocalcemia may develop; however, dose titration starting with 30 mg twice daily and increasing every 3 weeks did not result in hypocalcemia in a recent trial in PHPT [5]. It is also important to remember that drug interactions may occur related to strong inhibition of CYP2D6 and as a substrate of CYP3A4. The relatively high cost of cinacalcet may be an additional barrier for some patients.

Combination therapy with bisphosphonate and cinacalcet is an attractive option in PHPT as it would provide bone density improvement and calcium lowering. Neither agent alone can achieve this. Retrospective studies report benefits to both calcium and bone density with the combination but prospective trials or controlled trials are lacking [2].

Management

The lack of localization on imaging precluded considering an additional operation. This may be due to parathyromatosis which is often difficult to visualize (see Chap. 11). Her degree of hypercalcemia and symptoms were considered as reasons to initiate medical therapy, with a goal of normalizing her calcium and determining if that improved symptoms. She was advised about calcium and vitamin D intake and prescribed cinacalcet 30 mg once daily. This was titrated up to 30 mg twice daily and calcium levels normalized, and she reported improvement in her fatigue. Bisphosphonates were not initiated due to her near normal bone density.

Outcome

Two years later, she continues on cinacalcet and calcium remains normal although PTH is persistently mildly elevated. Bone density is unchanged. It is not clear how often to monitor bone density on cinacalcet therapy. She is at risk of bone loss as she enters the menopausal transition.

Clinical Pearls/Pitfalls
- Surgery remains the treatment of choice for PHPT patients needing treatment.
- Bisphosphonates, particularly alendronate, have been shown to improve bone density in PHPT, but may not be superior to surgery in improving bone density.
- Cinacalcet can lower or normalize serum calcium in PHPT but does not improve bone density.
- Combination therapy with both alendronate and cinacalcet may be attractive for patients with osteoporosis or high fracture risk and significant hypercalcemia.

Conflict of Interest All authors state that they have no conflicts of interest.

References

1. Richards ML, Thompson GB, Farley DR, Grant CS. Reoperative parathyroidectomy in 228 patients during the era of minimal-access surgery and intraoperative parathyroid hormone monitoring. Am J Surg [Comp Stud]. 2008;196(6):937–42. discussion 42-3.
2. Marcocci C, Bollerslev J, Khan AA, Shoback DM. Medical management of primary hyperparathyroidism: proceedings of the fourth International Workshop on the Management of Asymptomatic Primary Hyperparathyroidism. J Clin Endocrinol Metab [Consens Dev Conf]. 2014;99(10):3607–18.
3. Grey A, Lucas J, Horne A, Gamble G, Davidson JS, Reid IR. Vitamin D repletion in patients with primary hyperparathyroidism and coexistent vitamin D insufficiency. J Clin Endocrinol Metab [Res Support, Non-US Gov't]. 2005;90(4):2122–6.
4. Tournis S, Fakidari E, Dontas I, Liakou C, Antoniou J, Galanos A, et al. Effect of parathyroidectomy versus risedronate on volumetric bone mineral density and bone geometry at the tibia in

postmenopausal women with primary hyperparathyroidism. J Bone Miner Metab [Comp Stud Res Support, Non-US Gov't]. 2014;32(2):151–8.

5. Khan A, Bilezikian J, Bone H, Gurevich A, Lakatos P, Misiorowski W, et al. Cinacalcet normalizes serum calcium in a double-blind randomized, placebo-controlled study in patients with primary hyperparathyroidism with contraindications to surgery. Eur J Endocrinol [Multicenter Stud Randomized Control Trial Res Support, Non-US Gov't]. 2015;172(5):527–35.

6. Peacock M, Bilezikian JP, Bolognese MA, Borofsky M, Scumpia S, Sterling LR, et al. Cinacalcet HCl reduces hypercalcemia in primary hyperparathyroidism across a wide spectrum of disease severity. J Clin Endocrinol Metab [Clin Trial Multicenter Stud Randomized Control Trial Res Support, Non-US Gov't. 2011; 96(1):E9–18.

7. Brardi S, Cevenini G, Verdacchi T, Romano G, Ponchietti R. Use of cinacalcet in nephrolithiasis associated with normocalcemic or hypercalcemic primary hyperparathyroidism: results of a prospective randomized pilot study. Arch Ital Urol Androl [Randomized Control Trial]. 2015;87(1):66–71.

8. Marcocci C, Chanson P, Shoback D, Bilezikian J, Fernandez-Cruz L, Orgiazzi J, et al. Cinacalcet reduces serum calcium concentrations in patients with intractable primary hyperparathyroidism. J Clin Endocrinol Metab [Res Support, Non-US Gov't]. 2009;94(8):2766–72.

Chapter 14
Primary Hyperparathyroidism in Children and Adolescents

Hana Barbra Lo and Peter J. Tebben

Case Presentation

A 13-year-old previously healthy boy was referred for evaluation and treatment of hypercalcemia. His laboratory tests were calcium 11.5 mg/dL (9.6–10.6 mg/dL), parathyroid hormone (PTH) 121 pg/mL (15–65 pg/mL), phosphorus 3.7 mg/dL (4.0–5.2 mg/dL), and creatinine 0.7 mg/dL (0.4–0.8 mg/dL). He consumed approximately 1,000–1,200 mg of calcium daily through his diet. Growth and development had been normal. He had no history of fractures, nephrolithiasis, and no symptoms attributable to hypercalcemia. His urine calcium was elevated at 358 mg/day (5.8 mg/kg/day; nl – <4 mg/kg/day). X-ray of the

H.B. Lo, MD
Division of Endocrinology, Department of Pediatric and Adolescent Medicine, Mayo Clinic, Rochester, MN, USA

P.J. Tebben, MD (✉)
Division of Endocrinology, Department of Pediatric and Adolescent Medicine, Mayo Clinic, Rochester, MN, USA

Division of Endocrinology, Diabetes, Metabolism, and Nutrition, Department of Internal Medicine, Mayo College of Medicine, Mayo Clinic, Rochester, MN, USA
e-mail: tebben.peter@mayo.edu

A.E. Kearns, R.A. Wermers (eds.), *Hyperparathyroidism: A Clinical Casebook*, DOI 10.1007/978-3-319-25880-5_14, © Mayo Foundation for Medical Education and Research 2016 kidney, ureters, and bladder (KUB) did not identify occult kidney stone disease.

Laboratory assessment was performed due to a history of familial isolated primary hyperparathyroidism (FIPHPT). His father, older sister, and multiple additional paternal family members had undergone parathyroid surgery for PHPT. The underlying genetic cause for FIPHPT was unknown. There was no family history of pituitary disease, pancreatic/duodenal tumors, medullary thyroid cancer, adrenal tumors, or jaw tumors.

Six months later, his serum calcium increased to 12.5 mg/dL with a PTH of 163 pg/mL. He remained asymptomatic with no fractures or clinical renal disease. His calcitonin was normal as was his 24-h urine catecholamines and metanephrines. No jaw tumors were noted on physical exam.

Assessment and Diagnosis

Primary hyperparathyroidism (PHPT) is a commonly encountered endocrine disorder in adults, the incidence of which appeared to have increased after the introduction of automated serum calcium measurements in the 1970s, with another peak observed in the 1990s which coincided with the sharp increase in bone mineral density measurement. The overall incidence in adults reported from 1998 to 2010 was 50.4 per 100,000 person years [1, 2]. However, it is still a rare condition in infants and children with an incidence estimated at only 2–5 per 100,000 [3, 4]. Although some studies of children have suggested a male [5, 6] or female preponderance [3, 7], a recent review found no significant sexual predilection in children [4]. This is in contrast to the clear preponderance of disease in women in the adult population. Although PHPT is most commonly caused by a single adenoma in both children and adults, one study found that 31 % of children had familial disease which is in contrast to the small fraction of adults who have familial PHPT [3, 4]. As in adults, children with familial disease are much more likely to have parathyroid hyperplasia rather than a single adenoma. It is therefore critical to consider the family history when evaluating any child with PHPT.

Several germline gene defects have been identified that can lead to familial PHPT (Table 14.1) [4]. Neonatal severe hyperparathyroidism (NSPHPT) is a distinct form of PHPT caused by biallelic mutations in the *CASR* gene which encodes the calcium-sensing receptor, a G-protein-coupled receptor on the plasma membrane of parathyroid and renal tubule cells. Affected neonates may have severe metabolic bone disease and life-threatening hypercalcemia within the first few days of life, often requiring urgent intervention [4, 6, 8]. In contrast, heterozygous *CASR* mutations causing familial hypocalciuric hypercalcemia (FHH) typically lead to a mild and generally asymptomatic hypercalcemia [4, 8]. Multiple endocrine neoplasia type 1 (MEN1), a syndrome characterized by parathyroid, pancreatic, and pituitary tumors, is the most common cause of inherited PHPT. More than 90 % of MEN 1 patients will have PHPT, more commonly multiple adenomas or diffuse hyperplasia, and it is usually the first manifestation of the syndrome. Less common genetic syndromes causing PHPT include MEN2a, with 20–30 % of the patients developing PHPT, and hyperparathyroidism-jaw tumor (HPT-JT) syndrome, a rare autosomal dominant syndrome due to mutations in the *HRPT2* gene which is characterized by parathyroid adenomas and fibro-osseous lesions of the maxilla and mandible [4].

Elevated serum calcium with an elevated or inappropriately normal PTH is the hallmark biochemical feature that establishes the diagnosis of PHPT in children. This must be distinguished from secondary HPT that is commonly due to vitamin D and or calcium deficiency leading to elevated PTH concentrations with low-normal or low serum calcium levels. When evaluating a child with hypercalcemia, it is important to be aware that the normal ranges for serum calcium and phosphorus differ based on

Table 14.1 Clinical features of genetic syndromes associated with primary hyperparathyroidism

	MEN 1	MEN 2a	NSHPT/FHH	HPT-JT	FIHP
Clinical features	PHPT	PHPT	PHPT	PHPT	PHPT
	Pancreatic/duodenal tumors	Medullary thyroid carcinoma	Severe hypercalcemia in NSHPT	Fibro-osseous jaw tumors	
	Pituitary tumors (functioning and nonfunctioning)	Pheochromocytoma	Mild hypercalcemia in FHH	Uterine tumors	
	Skin findings (angiofibromas, collagenomas)		Low urine calcium	Renal tumors	
Genes affected	*MENIN*	*RET*	*CaSR*	*HRPT2/CDC73*	

MEN multiple endocrine neoplasia, *NSHPT* neonatal severe hyperparathyroidism, *FHH* familial hypocalciuric hypercalcemia, *HPT-JT* hyperparathyroidism-jaw tumor syndrome, *FIHP* familial isolated hyperparathyroidism, *PHPT* primary hyperparathyroidism age and gender (Table 14.2). Healthy infants and children have higher calcium and phosphorus concentrations compared to adults. This finding will influence the interpretation of laboratory studies, especially in children with mild calcium and parathyroid abnormalities. Urine calcium should also be interpreted with the age of the child in mind. Older children can often provide a 24-h urine sample in which case an upper limit of normal of 4 mg/kg/day can be applied. In infants and younger children, a calcium-to-creatine ratio on a spot urine sample can be used (Table 14.2). Some patients may also have hypophosphatemia, due to the action of PTH in the kidney and an elevated serum alkaline phosphatase, especially with documented bone involvement.

A recent review of the biochemical profile of children and adolescents with PHPT found a greater degree of hypercalcemia and hypercalciuria at presentation compared to adults despite similar parathyroid hormone concentrations. Furthermore, adenoma weight and alkaline phosphatase activity among age groups did not reveal significant difference. These observations suggest a possible greater sensitivity of target organs to PTH and an apparent decrease in the sensitivity of the parathyroid adenoma to negative feedback by calcium in young patients with PHPT [4, 9].

PHPT (especially sporadic) in children is associated with greater morbidity and end-organ damage at the time of diagnosis compared to adults. Most modern-day adult cohorts are asymptomatic and diagnosed incidentally [4, 9, 10], while as many as 79–91 % of children with PHPT present with symptoms attributable to the disease [3, 7, 11]. Another significant difference of juvenile compared with adult PHPT is the presence of end-organ damage at the time of diagnosis, the most common of which are renal and skeletal involvement [3, 11]. Bone disease, presenting as bone pain, radiographic evidence of osteopenia and osteolysis, diminished bone densitometry or fractures, occurs in about 43 % of children. Nephrolithiasis or nephrocalcinosis, at times leading to chronic kidney disease, is present in about 39 % [3, 4, 11].

Table 14.2 Age- and gender-appropriate normal values

	Normal values
Serum total calcium, males	
1–14 years	9.6–10.6 mg/dL
15–16 years	9.5–10.5 mg/dL
17–18 years	9.5–10.4 mg/dL
19–21 years	9.3–10.3 mg/dL
≥22 years	8.9–10.1 mg/dL
Serum total calcium, females	
1–11 years	9.6–10.6 mg/dL
12–14 years	9.5–10.4 mg/dL
15–18 years	9.1–10.3 mg/dL
≥19 years	8.9–10.1 mg/dL
Serum inorganic phosphorus, males	
1–4 years	4.3–5.4 mg/dL
5–13 years	3.7–5.4 mg/dL
14–15 years	3.5–5.3 mg/dL
16–17 years	3.1–4.7 mg/dL
≥18 years	2.5–4.5 mg/dL
Serum inorganic phosphorus, females	
1–7 years	4.3–5.4 mg/dL
8–13 years	4.0–5.2 mg/dL
14–15 years	3.5–4.9 mg/dL
16–17 years	3.1–4.7 mg/dL
≥18 years	2.5–4.5 mg/dL
Random urine calcium/creatinine ratio	
0–12 months	<2,100 mg/g
13–24 months	<450 mg/g
25 months–5 years	<350 mg/g
6–10 years	<300 mg/g
11–18 years	<260 mg/g
≥19 years	<220 mg/g

The normal values listed above were adapted from Mayo Medical Laboratories. Each laboratory may have different reference values

Nonspecific symptoms such as fatigue, poor appetite, weight loss, depression, hypertension, polyuria, polydipsia, abdominal pain, nausea, and vomiting may be the only manifestations of the disease or they may be associated with end-organ damage [3, 4, 11]. About 15 % of patients were asymptomatic at the time of diagnosis and were only discovered following an incidental finding of hypercalcemia [4]. This distinct clinical history of PHPT in children and adolescents may be attributed to several factors. Because routine biochemical screening is not performed as commonly in children as in adults, a degree of ascertainment bias may arise. As such, a diagnosis of PHPT is made only when the disease becomes symptomatic which is more reminiscent of PHPT in adults prior to the routine measurement of serum calcium [1, 12, 13]. Lack of specific symptoms may also lead to a delay in the appropriate diagnosis in many patients. The average delay occurring between the onset of symptoms and diagnosis ranges from 7.2 months to as long as 4.7 years in children [3, 7, 14]. Patients without renal symptoms had a longer duration of symptoms before a diagnosis of PHPT was secured. This significant delay in diagnosis unfortunately leads to more end-organ damage in this population.

Surgery is the only definitive treatment for PHPT and is the mainstay of management in pediatric patients. Currently, there are no existing guidelines on the management of asymptomatic children with PHPT. However, they have a higher potential to present with end-organ damage compared to adults [7]. Furthermore, a study that observed the natural history of asymptomatic adult patients who did not undergo surgery revealed progression of the disease in one third of the subjects over a 15-year follow-up [15]. Little information is available regarding the changes in skeletal and renal outcomes in children after parathyroidectomy. A single case report described a pronounced improvement in bone density after parathyroidectomy in a 16-year-old boy [16]. Resolution of renal stone disease has been reported in some children with persistent disease noted in others [7, 16]. The current consensus is that all asymptomatic adults less than 50 years of age should be considered for surgery [10]. It is therefore prudent to perform surgery in the pediatric population even if they have mild disease.

Surgical outcome in pediatric patients is generally excellent, with successful restoration of normal serum calcium in 94 % of cases [3]. This parallels previously reported success rates in adults [3, 17]. Short-term complications include postoperative transient hypocalcemia, musculoskeletal symptoms, and transient vocal cord paralysis. Long-term adverse events such as permanent vocal cord dysfunction or hypoparathyroidism are uncommon when performed by an experienced endocrine surgeon. Several reports have concluded that the incidence of complications, length of hospital stay, and cost correlates to surgeon volume, with superior outcomes observed among high-volume endocrine surgeons [18, 19].

Management

The patient underwent a parathyroid scan that revealed a clear left-sided parathyroid lesion (Fig. 14.1a). At surgery, a left superior 620 mg parathyroid gland was removed. Because of the family history, the left inferior parathyroid gland (30 mg) was also removed so as to avoid the need for future left neck exploration. Both glands were noted to be hypercellular. Four months after surgery, his serum calcium and parathyroid hormone concentrations were normal. Fifteen months after his initial surgery, he was found to have recurrent hyperparathyroidism with a serum calcium of 11.5 mg/dL, phosphorus of 2.7 mg/dL, creatinine of 0.8 mg/dL, and PTH of 79 pg/mL. His urine calcium was significantly elevated at 446 mg/day (7.3 mg/kg/day). Renal ultrasound did not identify nephrolithiasis or nephrocalcinosis.

His bone density measured by dual-energy x-ray absorptiometry (DXA) was normal. A parathyroid scan was obtained revealing a clear parathyroid lesion on the right (Fig. 14.1b). A second operation was undertaken and a 210 mg hypercellular right superior parathyroid gland was removed.

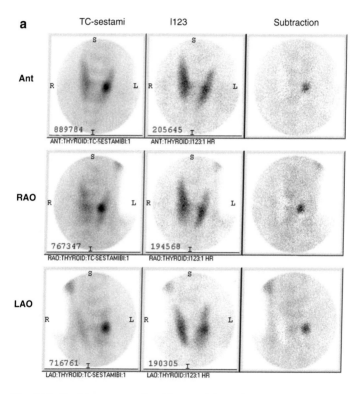

Fig. 14.1 Dual isotope parathyroid scan of the patient (**a**) at the time of diagnosis and (**b**) 15 months after the initial surgery

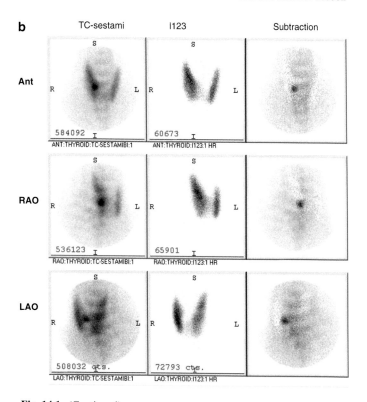

Fig. 14.1 (Continued)

Outcome

The patient recovered well from his second surgery without complications. He remains asymptomatic with normal serum calcium and parathyroid hormone concentrations 4 years after his second surgery.

Conflict of Interest All authors state that they have no conflicts of interest.

Clinical Pearls/Pitfalls
- Symptomatic disease with end-organ damage is common in children with PHPT.
- A detailed family history should be obtained for all children with PHPT and genetic disorders considered, especially in those with multi-gland disease/hyperplasia.
- Surgery should be undertaken by high-volume surgeons with experience in performing endocrine surgery in children.
- Age-appropriate normal ranges for serum calcium should be used when considering the diagnosis of hyperparathyroidism in children.

References

1. Wermers RA, Khosla S, Atkinson EJ, Achenbach SJ, Oberg AL, Grant CS, et al. Incidence of primary hyperparathyroidism in Rochester, Minnesota, 1993–2001: an update on the changing epidemiology of the disease. J Bone Miner Res. 2006;21(1):171–7.
2. Griebeler ML, Kearns AE, Ryu E, Hathcock MA, Melton 3rd LJ, Wermers RA. Secular trends in the incidence of primary hyperparathyroidism over five decades (1965–2010). Bone. 2015;73:1–7.
3. Kollars J, Zarroug AE, van Heerden J, Lteif A, Stavlo P, Suarez L, et al. Primary hyperparathyroidism in pediatric patients. Pediatrics. 2005;115(4):974–80.
4. Roizen J, Levine MA. Primary hyperparathyroidism in children and adolescents. J Chin Med Assoc: JCMA. 2012;75(9):425–34.
5. Hsu SC, Levine MA. Primary hyperparathyroidism in children and adolescents: the Johns Hopkins Children's Center experience 1984–2001. J Bone Mineral Res: Off J Am Soc Bone Mineral Res. 2002;17 Suppl 2:N44–50.
6. Loh KC, Duh QY, Shoback D, Gee L, Siperstein A, Clark OH. Clinical profile of primary hyperparathyroidism in adolescents and young adults. Clin Endocrinol. 1998;48(4):435–43.

7. Lawson ML, Miller SF, Ellis G, Filler RM, Kooh SW. Primary hyperparathyroidism in a paediatric hospital. QJM: Mon J Assoc Phys. 1996;89(12):921–32.
8. Pollak MR, Chou YH, Marx SJ, Steinmann B, Cole DE, Brandi ML, et al. Familial hypocalciuric hypercalcemia and neonatal severe hyperparathyroidism. Effects of mutant gene dosage on phenotype. J Clin Invest. 1994;93(3):1108–12.
9. Roizen J, Levine MA. A meta-analysis comparing the biochemistry of primary hyperparathyroidism in youths to the biochemistry of primary hyperparathyroidism in adults. J Clin Endocrinol Metab. 2014; 99(12):4555–64.
10. Bilezikian JP, Brandi ML, Eastell R, Silverberg SJ, Udelsman R, Marcocci C, et al. Guidelines for the management of asymptomatic primary hyperparathyroidism: summary statement from the Fourth International Workshop. J Clin Endocrinol Metab. 2014;99(10): 3561–9.
11. Harman CR, van Heerden JA, Farley DR, Grant CS, Thompson GB, Curlee K. Sporadic primary hyperparathyroidism in young patients: a separate disease entity? Arch Surg. 1999;134(6):651–5.
12. Keating Jr FR. Diagnosis of primary hyperparathyroidism. Clinical and laboratory aspects. JAMA. 1961;178:547–55.
13. Lafferty FW. Primary hyperparathyroidism. Changing clinical spectrum, prevalence of hypertension, and discriminant analysis of laboratory tests. Arch Intern Med. 1981;141(13):1761–6.
14. Rapaport D, Ziv Y, Rubin M, Huminer D, Dintsman M. Primary hyperparathyroidism in children. J Pediatr Surg. 1986;21(5):395–7.
15. Rubin MR, Bilezikian JP, McMahon DJ, Jacobs T, Shane E, Siris E, et al. The natural history of primary hyperparathyroidism with or without parathyroid surgery after 15 years. J Clin Endocrinol Metab. 2008;93(9):3462–70.
16. Vanstone MB, Udelsman RD, Cheng DW, Carpenter TO. Rapid correction of bone mass after parathyroidectomy in an adolescent with primary hyperparathyroidism. J Clin Endocrinol Metab. 2011;96(2): E347–50.
17. Marcocci C, Cetani F. Clinical practice. Primary hyperparathyroidism. N Engl J Med. 2011;365(25):2389–97.
18. Stavrakis AI, Ituarte PH, Ko CY, Yeh MW. Surgeon volume as a predictor of outcomes in inpatient and outpatient endocrine surgery. Surgery. 2007;142(6):887–99; discussion -99.
19. Tuggle CT, Roman SA, Wang TS, Boudourakis L, Thomas DC, Udelsman R, et al. Pediatric endocrine surgery: who is operating on our children? Surgery. 2008;144(6):869–77.

Chapter 15
Primary Hyperparathyroidism in Pregnancy

Haleigh James, Geoffrey B. Thompson, and Robert A. Wermers

Case Presentation

A 23-year-old pregnant woman was referred for management of primary hyperparathyroidism (PHPT) in the setting of multiple endocrine neoplasia type 1 (MEN1). Shortly after becoming pregnant, the patient's calcium was found to be 11.4 mg/dL. At the time of presentation, she was at 23-week gestation with the following laboratories: serum calcium, 10.2 mg/dL (nl, 8.9–10.1); phosphorus, 2.9 mg/dL (nl, 2.5–4.5); normal creatinine; and PTH, 45 pg/mL (nl, 15–65).

Her father and one of her three sisters also had MEN1, manifested by pancreatic neuroendocrine tumors, PHPT, and a pituitary tumor in her sister. She had been diagnosed with MEN1 by genetic testing (exon 10 Arg 527 stop) 6 years prior to pregnancy

H. James, MD • R.A. Wermers, MD (✉)
Division of Endocrinology, Diabetes, Metabolism, and Nutrition,
Department of Internal Medicine, Mayo College of Medicine,
Mayo Clinic, Rochester, MN, USA
e-mail: James.Haleigh@mayo.edu; wermers.robert@mayo.edu

G.B. Thompson, MD
Department of Surgery, Mayo College of Medicine, Mayo Clinic,
Rochester, MN, USA
e-mail: thompson.geoffrey@mayo.edu

A.E. Kearns, R.A. Wermers (eds.), *Hyperparathyroidism:
A Clinical Casebook*, DOI 10.1007/978-3-319-25880-5_15,
© Mayo Foundation for Medical Education and Research 2016

and was found to have associated PHPT. At that time, her serum total calcium was 10.5 mg/dL (nl, 9.1–10.3), phosphorus was 3.1 mg/dL (nl, 2.5–4.5), parathyroid hormone (PTH) level was 40 pg/mL, and creatinine was 0.7 mg/dL. Nuclear parathyroid scan showed mild focal increased uptake at the lower pole of the left thyroid lobe and posterior to the right thyroid lobe, consistent with small parathyroid adenomas. She had normal bone mineral density and no history of nephrolithiasis and denied symptoms of hypercalcemia such as polydipsia, polyuria, nausea, anorexia, constipation, pain, and neuropsychiatric changes, so the decision was made to forego surgery and monitor her serum calcium every 6 months.

Other studies done at that time of her initial diagnosis of MEN1 included a magnetic resonance imaging (MRI) of the brain with and without contrast with inclusion of a sella protocol, which was normal. A computed tomography (CT) scan of her abdomen with biphasic imaging of the pancreas was also unremarkable. She had normal gastrin, chromogranin A, human pancreatic polypeptide (HPP), glucagon, insulin-like growth factor 1 (IGF1), and prolactin levels.

Assessment and Diagnosis

Neck ultrasound showed a 7×3×5 mm hypoechoic oval nodule posterior to the right thyroid and a 4×2×3 mm nodule inferior to the left thyroid lobe, suggestive of possible parathyroid adenomas. An obstetrical ultrasound was normal with an estimated gestational age of 20 weeks and 6 days. Maternal fetal medicine recommended fetal heart rate monitoring before and immediately after surgery. They also suggested she be positioned with left lateral tilt during surgery to avoid vena cava compression and possible compromise to uterine blood flow. Finally, they felt her risk of preterm labor was remote and hence, did not recommend delaying surgery for antenatal steroids for fetal lung maturity.

MEN1 is an autosomal dominant condition caused by mutations in the tumor suppressor gene *MEN1*, which classically predisposes affected patients to tumors involving the parathyroid glands, anterior pituitary, and pancreatic islet cells. Carcinoid, adrenal cortical tumors, facial angiofibromas, collagenomas, and lipomatous tumors can also develop in MEN1. PHPT due to parathyroid adenomas is the most common manifestation of MEN1, occurring in 90 % of patients [1]. Compared to patients with sporadic PHPT, patients with MEN1-associated hyperparathyroidism usually present at an earlier age (second to fourth decade vs. sixth decade), have an equal male-to-female ratio (1:1 vs. 1:3), and have lower bone mineral density [2]. Many of these patients are diagnosed after hypercalcemia is noted incidentally, but they may also present with vague symptoms of hypercalcemia (polydipsia, polyuria, malaise, constipation, neuropsychiatric changes) or with nephrolithiasis [1].

It is recommended that patients with MEN1 be screened for hyperparathyroidism yearly with serum calcium and PTH measurements. While preoperative imaging is often performed in patients with sporadic PHPT to determine if patients are candidates for minimally invasive surgery [3], it is of limited benefit in MEN1 patients because multiple glands are usually affected and bilateral neck exploration is required regardless of imaging results in patients who undergo surgery [1]. Nonetheless, some surgeons prefer preoperative localization to aid with surgical planning, even in MEN1 patients.

PHPT in pregnancy is associated with several risks to both the mother and fetus. Maternal complications include hyperemesis, nephrolithiasis, mental status changes, muscle weakness, and rarely pancreatitis. Neonatal hypoparathyroidism, hypocalcemia, and even tetany may result from fetal PTH suppression in the setting of maternal hypercalcemia because calcium is transported across the placenta to the fetus. Hence, in pregnancies complicated by PHPT, the neonate should have monitoring of serum calcium, with awareness that hypoparathyroidism may not be present in the immediate post-partum period [4]. Also, formulas that are high in calcium and low in phosphate reduce the risk of hypocalcemia in these infants [5]. Low birth weight, preterm delivery, and miscarriage have also been associated with gestational PHPT, especially when hypercalcemia is pronounced [6, 7]. More recent data has shown that these complications are rare in the setting of mild maternal hypercalcemia (total serum calcium <11 mg/dL) [8].

The diagnosis of gestational PHPT is based on elevated serum calcium and PTH levels, just as in non-gestational PHPT. However, calcium is not routinely measured during pregnancy and gestational PHPT is often unrecognized [8]. Furthermore, several physiologic changes during pregnancy including hypoalbuminemia, increased glomerular filtration, transplacental transfer of calcium, and increased estrogen levels lower maternal serum calcium levels and may mask underlying PHPT [9]. PTH secretion is also suppressed during normal pregnancy due to increased intestinal calcium absorption and 1,25-dihydroxyvitamin D levels [10]. After biochemical confirmation, neck ultrasound is often utilized for preoperative localization in pregnant patients rather than nuclear or CT scans to eliminate risk to the fetus [7]. Thus, there would be no role for repeat nuclear parathyroid scan in this patient.

Management

The timing of parathyroid surgery in MEN1 patients with hyperparathyroidism is not well defined. Therefore, the indications for surgery (symptomatic or marked hypercalcemia, nephrolithiasis, osteoporosis, or renal insufficiency) used for patients with sporadic hyperparathyroidism [3] are often applied to MEN1 patients. When surgery is elected, it should consist of open bilateral neck exploration with cervical thymectomy and subtotal parathyroidectomy (at least 3.5 glands removed) or total parathyroidectomy with autologous transplantation performed by an experienced endocrine surgeon (see Chap. 9) [1].

In this case, management was altered by the patient's pregnancy. While clear treatment guidelines for PHPT in pregnancy are lacking, surgery is often performed to prevent the maternal and fetal risks described above. If observation of PHPT during pregnancy is considered, then adequate hydration combined with measurement of serum calcium and regular biophysical profiles of the fetus with ultrasound are recommended, with consideration of parathyroidectomy postpartum [10]. If surgery is recommended, then parathyroidectomy during the second trimester is preferred because organogenesis is complete and the risk of anesthesia-induced preterm delivery is lower than in the third trimester [7, 11]. Surgery was opted for in this case rather than continued monitoring of calcium, given her earlier serum calcium during pregnancy of 11.4 mg/dL. The patient underwent cervical exploration and excision of three enlarged parathyroid glands with autotransplantation of the left inferior parathyroid gland to the left anterior chest wall as a precaution. A fourth parathyroid gland was not found. Intraoperative PTH decreased from 58.8 to 14.5 pg/mL. Most pregnancies complicated by sporadic PHPT are due to a single parathyroid adenoma (89 %), which is similar to what is seen in nongestational PHPT [12].

Outcome

Postoperative calcium normalized to 9.2 mg/dL. The patient had no complications from the surgery, and she continued with regular obstetric cares.

Clinical Pearls/Pitfalls
- Patients with MEN1 should have serum calcium and PTH measured yearly to screen for PHPT because its prevalence is 90 % in this population.
- PHPT during pregnancy is associated with several risks to the mother (hyperemesis, nephrolithiasis, mental status changes, muscle weakness, and rarely pancreatitis) and fetus (neonatal hypoparathyroidism, hypocalcemia, tetany, low birth weight, preterm delivery, and miscarriage), especially when maternal total serum calcium is >11 mg/dL.
- If parathyroidectomy is opted for in a patient with gestational hyperparathyroidism, it should be performed in the second trimester.
- In gestational PHPT, neonates should have monitoring of serum calcium with awareness that hypoparathyroidism may not be present in the immediate postpartum period.

Conflict of Interest All authors state that they have no conflicts of interest.

References

1. Thakker RV, Newey PJ, Walls GV, Bilezikian J, Dralle H, Ebeling PR, et al. Clinical practice guidelines for multiple endocrine neoplasia type 1 (MEN1). J Clin Endocrinol Metab. 2012;97(9):2990–3011. Epub 2012/06/23.
2. Eller-Vainicher C, Chiodini I, Battista C, Viti R, Mascia ML, Massironi S, et al. Sporadic and MEN1-related primary hyperparathyroidism: differences in clinical expression and severity. J Bone Miner Res: Off J Am Soc Bone Miner Res. 2009;24(8):1404–10. Epub 2009/03/25.

3. Bilezikian JP, Brandi ML, Eastell R, Silverberg SJ, Udelsman R, Marcocci C, et al. Guidelines for the management of asymptomatic primary hyperparathyroidism: summary statement from the Fourth International Workshop. J Clin Endocrinol Metab. 2014;99(10):3561–9. Epub 2014/08/28.

4. Ip P. Neonatal convulsion revealing maternal hyperparathyroidism: an unusual case of late neonatal hypoparathyroidism. Arch Gynecol Obstet. 2003;268(3):227–9. Epub 2003/08/28.

5. Shangold MM, Dor N, Welt SI, Fleischman AR, Crenshaw Jr MC. Hyperparathyroidism and pregnancy: a review. Obstet Gynecol Surv. 1982;37(4):217–28. Epub 1982/04/01.

6. Norman J, Politz D, Politz L. Hyperparathyroidism during pregnancy and the effect of rising calcium on pregnancy loss: a call for earlier intervention. Clin Endocrinol (Oxf). 2009;71(1):104–9. Epub 2009/01/14.

7. Schnatz PF, Curry SL. Primary hyperparathyroidism in pregnancy: evidence-based management. Obstet Gynecol Surv. 2002;57(6):365–76. Epub 2002/07/26.

8. Hirsch D, Kopel V, Nadler V, Levy S, Toledano Y, Tsvetov G. Pregnancy outcomes in women with primary hyperparathyroidism. J Clin Endocrinol Metab. 2015;100(5):2115–22. Epub 2015/03/10.

9. Som M, Stroup JS. Primary hyperparathyroidism and pregnancy. Proc (Baylor Univ Med Cent). 2011;24(3):220–3. Epub 2011/07/09.

10. Kovacs CS. Parathyroid function and disease during pregnancy, lactation, and fetal/neonatal development. In: Bilezikian JP, Marcus R, Levine M, Marcocci C, Potts J, Silverberg S, editors. The parathyroids. 3rd ed. San Diego: Academic Press/Elsevier; 2014. p. 877–902.

11. Truong MT, Lalakea ML, Robbins P, Friduss M. Primary hyperparathyroidism in pregnancy: a case series and review. Laryngoscope. 2008;118(11):1966–9. Epub 2008/09/02.

12. Kelly TR. Primary hyperparathyroidism during pregnancy. Surgery. 1991;110(6):1028–33; discussion 33–4. Epub 1991/12/01.

Chapter 16
Primary Hyperparathyroidism: Association with Coexistent Secondary Causes of Hypercalcemia

Nicole M. Iñiguez-Ariza and Bart L. Clarke

Case Presentation

A 30-year-old female was referred for evaluation and management of hypercalcemia, first discovered during a routine clinical evaluation by her primary care physician. She was not taking any medications, but took vitamin D3 1000 international units once daily as a supplement. She did not take calcium supplementation. Her serum calcium was within the normal range 2 years ago. Her only symptom was fatigue. Her family history was unremarkable for hypercalcemia.

Her laboratory studies showed:

- Calcium 11.8 mg/dL (normal, 8.9–10.1 mg/dL)
- Phosphorus 3.0 mg/dL (normal, 2.5–4.5 mg/dL)
- Creatinine 0.8 mg/dL (normal, 0.6–1.1)

N.M. Iñiguez-Ariza, MD • B.L. Clarke, MD (✉)
Division of Endocrinology, Diabetes, Metabolism, and Nutrition,
Department of Internal Medicine, Mayo College of Medicine,
Mayo Clinic, Rochester, MN, USA
e-mail: clarke.bart@mayo.edu

A.E. Kearns, R.A. Wermers (eds.), *Hyperparathyroidism:*
A Clinical Casebook, DOI 10.1007/978-3-319-25880-5_16,
© Mayo Foundation for Medical Education and Research 2016

- Parathyroid hormone (PTH) 60 pg/mL (normal, 15–65 pg/mL)
- Albumin 4.0 g/dL (normal, 3.5–5.0)
- 25-hydroxyvitamin D 18 ng/mL (optimal, 25–50)
- 24-h urine calcium 317 mg/dL (normal, 20–275)

X-rays of her kidneys, ureters, and bladder showed nephrocalcinosis.

Her parathyroid sestamibi scan showed discordant uptake localizing to her right inferior parathyroid gland, without uptake elsewhere in her neck or chest.

Her age less than 50 years, serum calcium level greater than 11.0 mg/dL, evidence of kidney stones, and positive sestamibi scan were felt to represent indications for parathyroid surgery. She underwent elective right inferior parathyroidectomy. After removal of her right inferior parathyroid adenoma, her PTH value decreased by more than 50 % within 15 min of resection of her adenoma. During the first several days after surgery, her PTH unexpectedly continued to decrease to a nadir of 12 pg/mL, while her phosphorus level increased to 4.4 mg/dL, and her calcium level remained persistently increased at 10.7 mg/dL. Her pathology review confirmed that a right inferior parathyroid adenoma weighing 320 mg had been removed.

Her serum 1,25-dihydroxyvitamin D level was found to be increased after surgery. Her chest x ray was normal except for a few hilar lymph nodes. She felt better after surgery in spite of her persistently increased serum calcium level.

Assessment and Diagnosis

Persistent serum calcium elevation after successful parathyroid-ectomy, with a decreased PTH level, should raise the suspicion that a second cause of hypercalcemia is present. In this patient, her serum 1,25-dihydroxyvitamin D was increased despite the fact that her PTH level was decreased. Patients with primary hyperparathyroidism (PHPT) may have vitamin D deficiency, with decreased levels of serum 25-hydroxyvitamin D, and as a consequence, compensatory increase in serum 1,25-dihydroxyvitamin D due to PTH stimulation of renal 1-alpha-hydroxylase production of this form of vitamin D. Surgical cure of PHPT should result in a normal serum 1,25-dihydroxyvitamin D because PTH levels are normal.

The differential diagnosis of hypercalcemia is determined by the patient context. Outpatient hypercalcemia is most commonly caused by PHPT, whereas inpatient hypercalcemia is most commonly caused by malignancy. During hospitalization, supplementation with calcium, diets containing calcium, medications such as thiazide-type diuretics or lithium, immobilization, or dehydration can increase serum calcium levels.

Sporadic parathyroid adenomas causing PHPT are not usually diagnosed at her young age. The incidence of PHPT increases with age, with an increased incidence in women occurring between the ages of 50 and 60 years [1]. PHPT at her age may be due to familial genetic causes, which are more commonly associated with multi-gland hyperplasia.

The fact that she is less than 50 years old should raise the possibility of familial forms of PHPT, which are more common in younger patients, especially those less than 30 years of age. Familial forms of PHPT could also explain the persistence of hypercalcemia, since these forms may be associated with multi-gland parathyroid hyperplasia that may be missed at initial surgery. The fact that she had no family history of hyperparathyroidism, and had no other apparent endocrine disease, and that her PTH decreased significantly after surgery all argue against multi-gland disease. These findings suggest that her persistent hypercalcemia was not mediated by PTH after surgery and therefore less likely to be caused by a genetic mutation such as occurs in multiple endocrine neoplasia (MEN) type 1 or 2A, familial-isolated hyperparathyroidism, or hyperparathyroidism-jaw tumor syndromes. Nevertheless, genetic causes of hyperparathyroidism should always be considered in younger patients.

In the differential diagnosis of PHPT, familial hypocalciuric hypercalcemia (FHH) [2] is also a consideration. FHH is a rare autosomal dominant disease caused by inactivating mutations in the calcium-sensing receptor gene (*CASR*), leading to reduced parathyroid and renal tubular cell sensitivity to extracellular calcium, compensatory hyperparathyroidism, hypercalcemia, and hypocalciuria. Given that the patient's urine calcium was increased before surgery and that she had normal serum calcium documented several years earlier, it is highly unlikely that she has FHH, since this is a life-long benign condition that leads to hypercalcemia without complications, unlike what was described in the case presented.

Another possibility is that she could have hypercalcemia of malignancy, although the patient had no clinical evidence of cancer. The major causes of hypercalcemia due to malignancy [3] are humoral hypercalcemia of malignancy (HHM) in 80 % and osteolytic lesions due to metastatic bone disease in 20 %. Humoral hypercalcemia of malignancy involves secretion of an endocrine factor, most commonly parathyroid hormone-related peptide (PTHrP) overproduction by cancer cells. 1,25-dihydroxyvitamin D overproduction occurs in <1 %, while overproduction of PTH by cancer cells has only been described in case reports [4–11].

The most common cause of PTHrP-mediated hypercalcemia is solid organ malignancy, as confirmed by a recently published large case series. The diagnosis of PTHrP-mediated hypercalce-mia portended a poor prognosis in this study, with the median survival less than 2 months [12].

PTHrP was initially purified from human cancer cells in 1987 [13, 14]. The PTHrP gene encodes a 141-amino acid protein that shares 60–70 % sequence homology with PTH over the first 13 amino acids at the N-terminus [15]. Both PTH and PTHrP bind to a common PTH/PTHrP1 receptor (PTH/PTHrP1R) despite having structural differences [16, 17]. Hypercalcemia ensues only when PTHrP reaches a threshold concentration that surpasses the analogous actions of PTH [3]. PTHrP has equivalent actions to PTH in regulating bone resorption and renal calcium/phosphorus handling, via activation of osteoclastic bone resorption through increased osteoblast RANKL expression and via increased renal tubular calcium reabsorption and inhibition of phosphate reabsorption. However, PTHrP does not stimulate renal 1α-hydroxylase activity as much as PTH or increase serum 1,25-dihydroxyvitmain D levels as much [3, 18]. The discordant effects of PTH and PTHrP on 1,25-dihydroxyvitamin D production were confirmed in human-controlled clinical trials evaluating the effects of PTH (1-34) and PTHrP (1-36) infusions in healthy adults [19].

The clinical case described demonstrated increased levels of serum 1,25-dihydroxyvitamin D after surgery, which would not be expected in HHM caused by PTHrP, making HHM very unlikely. Asymptomatic skeletal metastasis would also be unusual in this setting. The rare hypercalcemia of malignancy caused by overproduction of 1,25-dihydroxyvitamin D occurs in less than 1 % of cases [3, 20] and is usually associated with hematologic malignancies such as Hodgkin or non-Hodgkin lymphoma, since immune cells of the lymphocyte and macrophage lineage normally produce a small amount of 1,25-dihydroxyvitamin D that acts as a local cytokine [21, 22].

In a patient with known malignancy who has increased or inappropriately normal PTH levels, it should be assumed that the patient has coexisting PHPT. Ectopic overproduction of PTH by tumor cells is highly unlikely, and patients with HHM caused by PTHrP overproduction have high calcium with low phosphorus levels as seen in PHPT, with PTH typically physiologically suppressed due to increased serum calcium.

In a prospective study [23] of consecutive patients with a first episode of hypercalcemia during an 18-month period, plasma PTHrP levels were increased in 82 % of patients with hypercalcemia due to malignancy. Hypercalcemia was attributable to parathyroid disease in 10 % of patients with malignancy. Median survival for patients with PHPT and coexisting malignancy was 13 months, compared to 3 months for those with hypercalcemia due to malignancy alone.

It should not be assumed that every patient with cancer and hypercalcemia must have a malignant etiology of their hypercalcemia. On the contrary, in a large series of cancer patients [24], nonmalignant causes of hypercalcemia in cancer patients were a frequent and neglected finding. Hypercalcemia was not due to cancer in 97 % (84/87) of the patients who were in complete remission from their cancer. Even in patients with active neoplastic disease, the number of patients whose hypercalcemia was not due to cancer was clinically relevant (115/555 = 20.5 %). In the 158 patients with PHPT, 92 patients were in complete remission, and 66 patients had active neoplastic disease. PHPT was the leading cause of non-cancer-related etiologies.

The most likely etiology of persistent hypercalcemia in the clinical case is granulomatous disease (Table 16.1), causing overproduction of 1,25-dihydroxyvitamin D by extra-renal 1α-hyroxylase activity. Of the various granulomatous diseases that can cause hypercalcemia, sarcoidosis, fungal disease, and tuberculosis are the most common in the USA. Therefore the next best step is to measure the angiotensin-converting enzyme (ACE) level and appropriate fungal serologies and to perform purified protein derivative (PPD) skin testing or Quantiferon measurement.

The patient was found to have a mildly increased ACE level of 60.9 units/L (normal, 8–53), negative fungal serologies, and negative PPD skin test. These findings were interpreted as suggesting the patient had coexisting sarcoidosis with her PHPT. ACE levels, although nonspecific, are useful in conjunction with other diagnostic procedures such as bronchoscopic needle biopsy, or biopsy of other accessible tissue such as bone marrow, with pathology showing noncaseating granulomas. The patient underwent bronchoscopic needle biopsy of one

Table 16.1 Causes of hypercalcemia

PTH excess	Malignancy	Non-PTH endocrine causes	Granulomatous disease	Medications	Miscellaneous
PHPT	HHM	Thyrotoxicosis	Sarcoidosis	Lithium	Immobilization
Parathyroid adenoma	PTHrP (80 %)	Adrenal insufficiency	Tuberculosis	Thiazides	Parenteral nutrition
Parathyroid carcinoma	$1,25-(OH)_2D$ (<1 %)	Pheochromocytoma	Coccidioidomycosis	Vitamin D intoxication	
Multiglandular hyperplasia as part of MEN syndromes (MEN1 and 2A)	PTH (<1 %)	VIPoma	Histoplasmosis	Excessive vitamin A	
	Bone mets/ local osteolysis (20 %): cytokines, local PTHrP	Acromegaly	Blastomycosis	Teriparatide	
			Berylliosis	Theophylline toxicity	
FIH			Leprosy	Milk-alkali syndrome	
HPT-JT			Crohn's disease		
FHH (UCCR <0.01)					
Tertiary HPT (renal failure)					

PHPT primary hyperparathyroidism, *MEN* multiple endocrine neoplasia, *FIH* familial-isolated hyperparathyroidism, *HPT-JT* hyperparathyroidism-jaw tumor syndrome, *FHH* familial hypocalciuric hypercalcemia, *UCCR* urinary calcium-creatinine clearance ratio, *HHM* humoral hypercalcemia of malignancy, *Mets* metastasis of her mediastinal lymph nodes, with her pathology report noting noncaseating granulomas, consistent with sarcoidosis.

A large health maintenance organization-based study estimated the annual incidence of sarcoidosis in Caucasians at 9.6 per 100,000 person-years and in African Americans at 35.5 per 100,000 person-years [25]. A Rochester Epidemiology Project population-based study in Rochester, Minnesota, estimated the annual incidence of sarcoidosis at 6.1 per 100,000 person-years [26]. Another Rochester Epidemiology Project population-based study indicated that the annual incidence of PHPT ranged between 15.8 and 129 per 100,000 person-years over 30 years, depending on the year incidence was assessed [1].

Patients may be suspected of having two coexisting causes of hypercalcemia, with PHPT often being the easier of the two to recognize. The first cases of coexisting PHPT and sarcoidosis were reported in 1958 [27]. Since then there have been mostly case reports or small case series of these coexisting disorders [28–30]. Evaluation of a recent large cohort of 50 patients with coexisting PHPT and sarcoidosis reported from the Mayo Clinic in Rochester, Minnesota [31], showed that patients with PHPT who had active sarcoidosis had higher serum ACE levels (60.9 ± 38.1 vs. 20.2 ± 14.0 units/L, P-value <0.0001), lower PTH levels (60 ± 24 vs. 96 ± 41 pg/mL, P-value 0.01), and lower phosphorus levels (2.7 ± 0.6 vs. 3.2 ± 0.5 mg/dL, P-value 0.02) than patients with PHPT alone. Reports of coexisting PHPT and secondary causes of hypercalcemia other than malignancy are less common.

Management

Recognition of the additional diagnosis of coexisting sarcoidosis, which was made evident after parathyroidectomy, led to treatment of the patient with prednisone 20 mg each day for 1 month, with rapid normalization of her serum calcium and a trend toward normalization of her serum phosphorus during her first week of treatment. Her prednisone was gradually tapered over the next 4 months, with persistently normal serum calcium.

Outcome

The patient was followed every 6 months for the next 5 years without recurrence of either her PHPT or sarcoidosis. Other patients may develop recurrence of either or both disorders in time.

Clinical Pearls/Pitfalls
- Age, gender, and magnitude of hypercalcemia should be considered, as well as variation in serum PTH, calcium, phosphorus, and 1,25-dihydroxyvitamin D levels and patient context, when assessing possible etiologies of hypercalcemia.
- When coexisting causes of hypercalcemia are suspected or known to be present, classical findings of PHPT should not be expected.
- When faced with the possibility of coexisting causes of hypercalcemia, the clinical approach should be tailored to the patient after analyzing all available laboratory and imaging data.
- Patients presenting with hypercalcemia may have several causes contributing to their hypercalcemia. Dehydration, renal insufficiency, or vitamin D or A excess, in addition to increased PTH or granulomatous overproduction of 1,25-dihydroxyvitamin D, may all contribute to hypercalcemia in the same patient. The challenge for the clinician is to tease out the major cause or causes of hypercalcemia.
- Consideration of the complete differential diagnosis of hypercalcemia in each case is important since different causes of increased serum calcium levels are treated in distinctive ways.

Conflict of Interest All authors state that they have no conflicts of interest.

References

1. Wermers RA, Khosla S, Atkinson EJ, Achenbach SJ, Oberg AL, Grant CS, et al. Incidence of primary hyperparathyroidism in Rochester, Minnesota, 1993–2001: an update on the changing epidemiology of the disease. J Bone Miner Res. 2006;21:171–7.
2. Christensen SE, Nissen PH, Vestergaard P, Mosekilde L. Familial hypocalciuric hypercalcaemia: a review. Curr Opin Endocrinol. 2011;18:359–70.
3. Clines GA. Mechanisms and treatment of hypercalcemia of malignancy. Curr Opin Endocrinol. 2011;18:339–46.
4. Iguchi H, Miyagi C, Tomita K, Kawauchi S, Nozuka Y, Tsuneyoshi M, et al. Hypercalcemia caused by ectopic production of parathyroid hormone in a patient with papillary adenocarcinoma of the thyroid gland. J Clin Endocrinol Metab. 1998;83(8):2653–7.
5. Nielsen PK, Rasmussen AK, Feldt-Rasmussen U, Brandt M, Christensen L, Olgaard K. Ectopic production of intact parathyroid hormone by a squamous cell lung carcinoma in vivo and in vitro. J Clin Endocrinol Metab. 1996;81:3793–6.
6. Nussbaum SR, Gaz RD, Arnold A. Hypercalcemia and ectopic secretion of parathyroid hormone by an ovarian carcinoma with rearrangement of the gene for parathyroid hormone. N Engl J Med. 1990;323:1324–8.
7. Rizzoli R, Pache JC, Didierjean L, Burger A, Bonjour JP. A thymoma as a cause of true ectopic hyperparathyroidism. J Clin Endocrinol Metab. 1994;79:912–5.
8. Strewler GJ, Budayr AA, Clark OH, Nissenson RA. Production of parathyroid hormone by a malignant nonparathyroid tumor in a hypercalcemic patient. J Clin Endocrinol Metab. 1993;76:1373–5.
9. VanHouten JN, Yu N, Rimm D, Dotto J, Arnold A, Wysolmerski JJ, et al. Hypercalcemia of malignancy due to ectopic transactivation of the parathyroid hormone gene. J Clin Endocrinol Metab. 2006;91:580–3.
10. Wong K, Tsuda S, Mukai R, Sumida K, Arakaki R. Parathyroid hormone expression in a patient with metastatic nasopharyngeal rhabdomyosarcoma and hypercalcemia. Endocrine. 2005;27:83–6.

11. Yoshimoto K, Yamasaki R, Sakai H, Tezuka U, Takahashi M, Iizuka M, et al. Ectopic production of parathyroid hormone by small cell lung cancer in a patient with hypercalcemia. J Clin Endocrinol Metab. 1989;68:976–81.

12. Donovan PJ, Achong N, Griffin K, Galligan J, Pretorius CJ, McLeod DS. PTHrP-mediated hypercalcemia: causes and survival in 138 patients. J Clin Endocrinol Metab. 2015;100:2024–9.

13. Moseley JM, Kubota M, Diefenbach-Jagger H, Wettenhall RE, Kemp BE, Suva LJ, et al. Parathyroid hormone-related protein purified from a human lung cancer cell line. Proc Natl Acad Sci U S A. 1987;84:5048–52.

14. Strewler GJ, Stern PH, Jacobs JW, Eveloff J, Klein RF, Leung SC, et al. Parathyroid hormonelike protein from human renal carcinoma cells. Structural and functional homology with parathyroid hormone. J Clin Invest. 1987;80:1803–7.

15. Suva LJ, Winslow GA, Wettenhall RE, Hammonds RG, Moseley JM, Diefenbach-Jagger H, et al. A parathyroid hormone-related protein implicated in malignant hypercalcemia: cloning and expression. Science. 1987;237:893–6.

16. Abou-Samra AB, Juppner H, Force T, Freeman MW, Kong XF, Schipani E, et al. Expression cloning of a common receptor for parathyroid hormone and parathyroid hormone-related peptide from rat osteoblast-like cells: a single receptor stimulates intracellular accumulation of both cAMP and inositol trisphosphates and increases intracellular free calcium. Proc Natl Acad Sci U S A. 1992;89:2732–6.

17. Pioszak AA, Parker NR, Gardella TJ, Xu HE. Structural basis for parathyroid hormone-related protein binding to the parathyroid hormone receptor and design of conformation-selective peptides. J Biol Chem. 2009;284:28382–91.

18. Dean T, Vilardaga JP, Potts Jr JT, Gardella TJ. Altered selectivity of parathyroid hormone (PTH) and PTH-related protein (PTHrP) for distinct conformations of the PTH/PTHrP receptor. Mol Endocrinol. 2008;22:156–66.

19. Horwitz MJ, Tedesco MB, Sereika SM, Syed MA, Garcia-Ocana A, Bisello A, et al. Continuous PTH and PTHrP infusion causes suppression of bone formation and discordant effects on 1,25(OH)2 vitamin D. J Bone Miner Res. 2005;20:1792–803.

20. Stewart AF. Clinical practice. Hypercalcemia associated with cancer. N Engl J Med. 2005;352:373–9.

21. Edfeldt K, Liu PT, Chun R, Fabri M, Schenk M, Wheelwright M, et al. T-cell cytokines differentially control human monocyte antimicrobial

responses by regulating vitamin D metabolism. Proc Natl Acad Sci U S A. 2010;107:22593–8.

22. Nelson CD, Reinhardt TA, Beitz DC, Lippolis JD. In vivo activation of the intracrine vitamin D pathway in innate immune cells and mammary tissue during a bacterial infection. PLoS One. 2010;5:e15469.

23. Walls J, Ratcliffe WA, Howell A, Bundred NJ. Parathyroid hormone and parathyroid hormone-related protein in the investigation of hypercalcaemia in two hospital populations. Clin Endocrinol (Oxf). 1994;41:407–13.

24. Soyfoo MS, Brenner K, Paesmans M, Body JJ. Non-malignant causes of hypercalcemia in cancer patients: a frequent and neglected occurrence. Support Care Cancer. 2013;21:1415–9.

25. Rybicki BA, Major M, Popovich Jr J, Maliarik MJ, Iannuzzi MC. Racial differences in sarcoidosis incidence: a 5-year study in a health maintenance organization. Am J Epidemiol. 1997;145:234–41.

26. Henke CE, Henke G, Elveback LR, Beard CM, Ballard DJ, Kurland LT. The epidemiology of sarcoidosis in Rochester, Minnesota: a population-based study of incidence and survival. Am J Epidemiol. 1986;123:840–5.

27. Snapper I, Yarvis JJ, Freund HR, Goldberg AF. Hyperparathyroidism in identical twins, one of whom suffered concomitantly of Boeck's sarcoidosis. Metabolism. 1958;7:671–80.

28. Balasanthiran A, Sandler B, Amonoo-Kuofi K, Swamy R, Kaniyur S, Kaplan F. Sarcoid granulomas in the parathyroid gland – a case of dual pathology: hypercalcaemia due to a parathyroid adenoma and coexistent sarcoidosis with granulomas located within the parathyroid adenoma and thyroid gland. Endocr J. 2010;57:603–7.

29. Hassan S, Amer S, Swamy V, Rao S. Sarcoidosis and primary hyperparathyroidism simultaneously occurring in a hypercalcemic patient. Indian J Endocrinol Metab. 2012;16:1062–3.

30. Yoshida T, Iwasaki Y, Kagawa T, Sasaoka A, Horino T, Morita T, et al. Coexisting primary hyperparathyroidism and sarcoidosis in a patient with severe hypercalcemia. Endocr J. 2008;55:391–5.

31. Lim V, Clarke BL. Coexisting primary hyperparathyroidism and sarcoidosis cause increased angiotensin-converting enzyme and decreased parathyroid hormone and phosphate levels. J Clin Endocrinol Metab. 2013;98:1939–45.

Chapter 17
Medication Considerations in Hypercalcemia and Hyperparathyroidism

Robert A. Wermers and Marcio L. Griebeler

Case Presentation

An 82-year-old female is referred for evaluation of hypercalcemia, with a serum calcium of 11.7 mg/dL (nl, 8.9–10.1) that was identified on lab work 1 month prior after she complained of increasing fatigue over the last 2 months. Subsequent laboratory testing identified the following: serum calcium – 10.8 mg/dL and phosphorus – 3.7 mg/dL (nl, 2.5–4.5) with at concomitant PTH of 48 pg/mL (nl, 15–50). Previous calcium measurements were noted to be normal, but more recently when checked, were high normal. Further laboratory studies that were done and normal included TSH, complete blood count, serum protein electrophoresis, serum creatinine, and 25-hydroxyvitamin D. Her

R.A. Wermers, MD (✉)
Division of Endocrinology, Diabetes, Metabolism, and Nutrition,
Department of Internal Medicine, Mayo College of Medicine,
Mayo Clinic, Rochester, MN, USA
e-mail: wermers.robert@mayo.edu

M.L. Griebeler, MD
Department of Internal Medicine, Sanford University of South Dakota
Medical Center, Sioux Falls, SD, USA

A.E. Kearns, R.A. Wermers (eds.), *Hyperparathyroidism:*   149
A Clinical Casebook, DOI 10.1007/978-3-319-25880-5_17,
© Mayo Foundation for Medical Education and Research 2016

medications of note included one calcium carbonate daily (600 mg elemental calcium per tablet), one multivitamin per day, and hydrochlorothiazide 25 mg one daily for hypertension. Her estimated daily dietary calcium intake was 600 mg per day. She denied a history of external beam radiation treatments to her head or neck, and there was no family history of primary hyperparathyroidism (PHPT) or hypercalcemia, familial endocrine syndromes, or hip fractures.

She denied a history of nephrolithiasis or fragility fractures. Her dual-energy X-ray absorptiometry (DXA) bone mineral density (BMD) revealed a non-dominant left one-third radius T-score of – 0.5, worst femur neck T-score of – 2.0, and lumbar spine T-score of – 1.0. The hip and spine had declined 6.2 % and 4.7 %, respectively, both greater than the least significant change, from the previous measure done approximately 6.5 years previously. Her physical examination revealed a height of 157.6 cm, weight of 85.1 kg, and blood pressure of 136/64 but was otherwise unremarkable.

Assessment and Diagnosis

The patient's lab work is consistent with primary hyperparathyroidism (PHPT). However, thiazide diuretics can also be associated with hypercalcemia [1]. Increased renal tubular reabsorption of calcium resulting in reduced urine calcium excretion is the most likely explanation for hypercalcemia associated with thiazide diuretics [2–4]. A mean increase of 0.8 mg/dL in albumin-adjusted serum calcium level is seen with thiazide use. Serum calcium concentrations are increased independently of PTH [5]. However, the increase in renal tubular calcium resorption and serum calcium is no longer observed after 2 years of therapy [6]. Upon review of the patient's medical record, she had been on hydrochlorothiazide for more than 10 years, making it unlikely that thiazide use was the primary cause of her hypercalcemia. It is estimated that approximately two-thirds of patients with thiazide-associated hypercalcemia have underlying PHPT, based on the persistence of hypercalcemia after discontinuation of the thiazide [1]. Additional factors favoring PHPT in thiazide-associated hypercalcemia include higher serum calcium and PTH levels at diagnosis [1].

Several other medications have effects on PTH and serum calcium that should be considered when evaluating patients with PHPT. In women with PHPT, estrogen and raloxifene lower serum total calcium, but PTH levels do not change significantly [7, 8]. PTH secretion can also be modified by calcium [9] and vitamin D supplements [10] in PHPT subjects. Lithium has been associated with hypercalcemia as well as parathyroid hyperplasia and adenomas [11].

There are a number of other commonly used medications that can influence PTH and calcium measurements in patients without PHPT. Aromatase inhibitors such as letrozole have been associated with a reduction in PTH in postmenopausal women likely related to efflux of calcium from the skeleton with lower estrogen levels [12]. On the other hand, there is a trend toward an increase in PTH with estrogen treatment in postmenopausal women without PHPT likely related to a reduction in skeletal calcium release [13, 14]. Similarly, antiresorptive osteoporosis therapies such as denosumab [15] and potent bisphosphonates [16–18] can also be associated with an increase in PTH and reductions in serum calcium levels. Teriparatide, rhPTH (1–34), can lead to mild elevations of serum calcium in osteoporotic subjects, but are generally not clinically meaningful [19]. In addition, the timing of the serum calcium measurement after the teriparatide is critical, such that measures done >16 h post-dose are unlikely to be elevated [19, 20]. Several antihypertensive agents have effects on PTH secretion without significant effects on serum calcium including loop diuretics and calcium channel blockers which have been associated with an increased PTH

[21, 22], whereas renin-angiotensin-aldosterone system inhibi-tors have been associated with a lower PTH [22]. Finally, anti-retroviral therapy for HIV-1 infection which includes tenofovir disoproxil fumarate (TDF) is also associated with increased PTH and excess bone loss [23].

Management

The patient followed-up 3 months after discontinuation of hydrochlorothiazide and her serum calcium and phosphorus were 11 mg/dL and 3.6 mg/dL, respectively, with a PTH of 70 pg/mL, consistent with PHPT. Long-term discontinuation of hydrochlorothiazide may not be necessary in patients with thiazide-associated hypercalcemia since serious sequelae related to hyper-calcemia in these patients despite continued use are rare [1]. However, she remained off of hydrochlorothiazide and opted to observe after a discussion about the risks and benefits of para-thyroid surgery. She did have a 10-year probability of major osteoporotic and hip fracture risk, as calculated by WHO Fracture Risk Assessment Tool (FRAX®), of 15 % and 4 %, respectively. Hence, after a discussion of risks and benefits of alendronate therapy, she decided to initiate treatment. She was advised to continue her current calcium intake and avoid falls.

Outcome

The patient remained clinically stable over years of follow-up. Her maximum serum calcium level, 5 years after her initial elevation, was 11.2 mg/dL. However, she had intermittently high normal calcium measurements as well. Her last measured serum calcium was 10.1 mg/dL at 7 years after her diagnosis of PHPT. Her PTH was periodically measured and was generally

1.5-fold elevated. Her primary provider discontinued alendronate after 6.5 years of treatment. The patient fell, suffered an acetabular fracture, and died shortly thereafter at 90 years of age, 8 years after her diagnosis of PHPT.

Clinical Pearls/Pitfalls

- Approximately two-third patients with thiazide-associated hypercalcemia have underlying PHPT.
- After 2 years of thiazide use, the increase in renal tubular calcium resorption and serum calcium is no longer observed.
- Many commonly used medications can influence the calcium and PTH measurement in patients with PHPT, including estrogen, raloxifene, calcium, and vitamin D.
- A number of other commonly used medications can influence PTH and calcium measurements in patients without PHPT including numerous antihypertensive agents, aromatase inhibitors, estrogen, tenofovir, and several osteoporosis therapies.
- In patients with PHPT and increased fracture risk, who opt for observation rather than parathyroidectomy, consider treatment with bisphosphonates.

Conflict of Interest All authors state that they have no conflicts of interest.

References

1. Wermers RA, Kearns AE, Jenkins GD, Melton 3rd LJ. Incidence and clinical spectrum of thiazide-associated hypercalcemia. Am J Med. 2007;120:911 e919–915.
2. Brickman AS, Massry SG, Coburn JW. Changes in serum and urinary calcium during treatment with hydrochlorothiazide: studies on mechanisms. J Clin Invest. 1972;51:945–54.

3. Grieff M, Bushinsky DA. Diuretics and disorders of calcium homeostasis. Semin Nephrol. 2011;31:535–41.
4. Middler S, Pak CY, Murad F, Bartter FC. Thiazide diuretics and calcium metabolism. Metabolism. 1973;22:139–46.
5. Rejnmark L, Vestergaard P, Heickendorff L, Andreasen F, Mosekilde L.
   Loop diuretics alter the diurnal rhythm of endogenous parathyroid
   hormone secretion. A randomized-controlled study on the effects of
   loop- and thiazide-diuretics on the diurnal rhythms of calcitropic hor-
   mones and biochemical bone markers in postmenopausal women. Eur
   J Clin Invest. 2001;31:764–72.
6. Bolland MJ, Ames RW, Horne AM, Orr-Walker BJ, Gamble GD, Reid
   IR. The effect of treatment with a thiazide diuretic for 4 years on bone
   density in normal postmenopausal women. Osteoporos Int. 2007;18:
   479–86.
7. Marcus R, Madvig P, Crim M, Pont A, Kosek J. Conjugated estrogens
   in the treatment of postmenopausal women with hyperparathyroidism.
   Ann Intern Med. 1984;100:633–40.
8. Rubin MR, Lee KH, McMahon DJ, Silverberg SJ. Raloxifene lowers
   serum calcium and markers of bone turnover in postmenopausal
   women with primary hyperparathyroidism. J Clin Endocrinol Metab.
   2003;88:1174–8.
9. Tohme JF, Bilezikian JP, Clemens TL, Silverberg SJ, Shane E,
   Lindsay R. Suppression of parathyroid hormone secretion with oral
   calcium in normal subjects and patients with primary hyperparathyroidism. J Clin Endocrinol Metab. 1990;70:951–6.
10. Grey A, Lucas J, Horne A, Gamble G, Davidson JS, Reid IR. Vitamin
    D repletion in patients with primary hyperparathyroidism and coexistent
    vitamin D insufficiency. J Clin Endocrinol Metab. 2005;90:2122–6.
11. Mallette LE, Eichhorn E. Effects of lithium carbonate on human cal-
    cium metabolism. Arch Intern Med. 1986;146:770–6.
12. Heshmati HM, Khosla S, Robins SP, O'Fallon WM, Melton 3rd LJ,
    Riggs BL. Role of low levels of endogenous estrogen in regulation of
    bone resorption in late postmenopausal women. J Bone Miner Res.
    2002;17:172–8.
13. Khosla S, Melton 3rd LJ, Riggs BL. The unitary model for estrogen
    deficiency and the pathogenesis of osteoporosis: is a revision needed?
    J Bone Miner Res. 2011;26:441–51.
14. Lufkin EG, Wahner HW, O'Fallon WM, et al. Treatment of postmeno-
    pausal osteoporosis with transdermal estrogen. Ann Intern Med.
    1992;117:1–9.
15. Bekker PJ, Holloway DL, Rasmussen AS, et al. A single-dose placebo-
    controlled study of AMG 162, a fully human monoclonal antibody to

RANKL, in postmenopausal women. J Bone Miner Res. 2004;19: 1059–66.

16. Adami S, Mian M, Bertoldo F, et al. Regulation of calcium-parathyroid hormone feedback in primary hyperparathyroidism: effects of bisphosphonate treatment. Clin Endocrinol. 1990;33:391–7.

17. Generali D, Dovio A, Tampellini M, et al. Changes of bone turnover markers and serum PTH after night or morning administration of zoledronic acid in breast cancer patients with bone metastases. Br J Cancer. 2008;98:1753–8.

18. Greenspan SL, Holland S, Maitland-Ramsey L, et al. Alendronate stimulation of nocturnal parathyroid hormone secretion: a mechanism to explain the continued improvement in bone mineral density accompanying alendronate therapy. Proc Assoc Am Physicians. 1996;108: 230–8.

19. Wermers RA, Recknor CP, Cosman F, Xie L, Glass EV, Krege JH. Effects of teriparatide on serum calcium in postmenopausal women with osteoporosis previously treated with raloxifene or alendronate. Osteoporosis Int. 2008;19:1055–65.

20. Krege JH, Donley DW, Marcus R. Teriparatide, osteoporosis, calcium, and vitamin D. N Engl J Med. 2005;353:634–5; author reply 634–5.

21. Rejnmark L, Vestergaard P, Pedersen AR, Heickendorff L, Andreasen F, Mosekilde L. Dose-effect relations of loop- and thiazide-diuretics on calcium homeostasis: a randomized, double-blinded Latin-square multiple cross-over study in postmenopausal osteopenic women. Eur J Clin Invest. 2003;33:41–50.

22. Brown J, de Boer IH, Robinson-Cohen C, et al. Aldosterone, parathyroid hormone, and the use of renin-angiotensin-aldosterone system inhibitors: the multi-ethnic study of atherosclerosis. J Clin Endocrinol Metab. 2015;100:490–9.

23. Overton ET, Chan ES, Brown TT, Tebas P, McComsey GA, Melbourne KM, Napoli A, Hardin WR, Ribaudo HJ, Yin MT. Vitamin D and calcium attenuate bone loss with antiretroviral therapy initiation. Ann Intern Med. 2015;162:815–24.

Chapter 18
Normocalcemic Primary Hyperparathyroidism

Jad G. Sfeir and Matthew T. Drake

Case Presentation

A 54-year-old female with a prior history notable only for two episodes of nephrolithiasis which had occurred 8 years previously was referred by her primary care provider who noted that the patient had an elevated parathyroid hormone (PTH) level. On evaluation, the patient denied any current neurologic or gastrointestinal complaints and was otherwise healthy. She was not taking any regular calcium supplements but did take ergocalciferol 50,000 IU once monthly. Her biochemical testing (Table 18.1) revealed normal serum calcium and elevated PTH. Dual-energy X-ray absorptiometry obtained 3 months previously had revealed normal bone mineral density.

J.G. Sfeir, MD • M.T. Drake, MD, PhD (✉)
Division of Endocrinology, Diabetes, Metabolism, and Nutrition,
Department of Internal Medicine, Mayo College of Medicine,
Mayo Clinic, Rochester, MN, USA
e-mail: jgsfeir@gmail.com; drake.matthew@mayo.edu

A.E. Kearns, R.A. Wermers (eds.), *Hyperparathyroidism:*
A Clinical Casebook, DOI 10.1007/978-3-319-25880-5_18,
© Mayo Foundation for Medical Education and Research 2016

Table 18.1 Patient's laboratory data at time of presentation and when assessed 3 months previously

Analyte	3 months previously	Current presentation	Reference range
Calcium	9.5	9.6	8.9–10.1 mg/dL
Phosphorus	1.9	2.0	2.5–4.5 mg/dL
Creatinine	0.5	0.7	0.6–1.1 mg/dL
Parathyroid hormone	103.5	81.2	15–65 pg/mL
25-hydroxyvitamin D	21	25.3	20–50 ng/mL
1,25-dihydroxyvitamin D	–	71	18–78 pg/mL
TSH	0.97	–	0.3–4.2 mIU/L
24-h urinary calcium	280	390	25–300 mg/24 h
24-h urinary phosphorus	–	1347 mg	<1100 mg/24 h

PTH parathyroid hormone, *TSH* thyroid-stimulating hormone

Review of her records indicated a highest calcium level (10.5 mg/dL) approximately 6 months prior to the current evaluation, when she had been taking up to ten tablets of calcium carbonate per day (1000 mg) for self-management of heartburn and reflux. This had been stopped due to the elevated calcium value, and she has not been maintained on any calcium supplementation since that time.

Assessment and Diagnosis

Primary hyperparathyroidism (PHPT) has been well recognized as a very common endocrine disorder with well-characterized diagnostic and prognostic features since the early 1970s when serum metabolic panels were introduced for routine screening that could detect hypercalcemia in otherwise asymptomatic patients. Over the past two decades, normocalcemic primary hyperparathyroidism (NPHPT) has been identified as a new subset of this disease in what Silverberg and Bilezikian referred to as a "forme fruste" of PHPT, identified primarily in patients referred for evaluation of low bone mass or less commonly nephrolithiasis [1].

NPHPT is defined by elevated PTH levels that occur concomitant with normal albumin-corrected serum calcium levels, after exclusion of secondary hyperparathyroidism [2] as an etiology. In contrast to PHPT patients in whom normal calcium levels may occur intermittently, patients with NPHPT are consistently normocalcemic on repeated evaluations. As discussed below, some patients may progress to overt hypercalcemia; such patients would then be considered to have progressed to PHPT [3].

NPHPT should be first suspected in patients having an elevated PTH level with consistently normal albumin-corrected serum calcium levels. However, several nuances to these diagnostic features are to be noted.

First, several sources suggest ensuring normal ionized calcium as well [4, 5]. Up to 10 % of patients with PHPT can have normal total serum calcium and elevated ionized calcium levels [6]. Obtaining ionized calcium levels, however, can be labor intensive and may not be readily available in the outpatient setting. Correcting for hypoalbuminemia eliminates the major difference that may occur between total serum calcium and ionized calcium.

Second, exclusion of secondary causes of hyperparathyroidism is essential to the diagnosis of NPHPT. The most important secondary causes are listed in Table 18.2.

Most notably, serum 25-hydroxyvitamin D levels below 30 ng/mL may cause increased PTH levels. Whereas some authors have used a cut point of 20 ng/mL to exclude hypovitaminosis D as a driving force for increased PTH levels, other authors have demonstrated that 25-hydroxyvitamin D levels between 20 and 30 may affect PTH levels [7, 8]. Furthermore, PTH levels have been shown to begin to rise when GFR falls below 60 mL/min and continue to increase as kidney function worsens [9, 10]. Several medications have also been associated

Table 18.2 Causes of secondary hyperparathyroidism

Causes of secondary hyperparathyroidism
Hypovitaminosis D
Decreased glomerular filtration rate
Thyroid disease
Hypercalciuria
Malabsorptive diseases (e.g., celiac disease)
Liver and pancreatic diseases
Other bone diseases (e.g., Paget's disease of bone)
Medications (e.g., thiazide diuretics, lithium, etc.)

with elevated PTH levels, most notably thiazide diuretics and lithium, but also estrogens, bisphosphonates, denosumab, and anticonvulsants [4].

Initial observations of NPHPT were based on populations referred to metabolic bone clinics for the evaluation of low bone mass and therefore tended to overestimate disease prevalence. Several attempts have been made to evaluate the prevalence of NPHPT in population-based cohorts. Reproducibility and generalizability of these numbers, however, appear to be limited as studies have tended to differ in gender distribution, geographic location, and efforts to exclude cases of secondary hyperparathyroidism.

In a survey of 5202 postmenopausal women in Sweden between the ages of 55 and 75, an estimated 0.5 % had elevated PTH levels with normal serum calcium values. Although this cohort did not exclude secondary etiologies of hyperparathyroidism, most cases of NPHPT were confirmed by surgical pathology [11].

Based on the NHANES data, Misra et al. found that 1 % of men and women aged greater than 45 years had PTH levels of 65 pg/mL or higher in addition to normal albumin-corrected serum calcium values. Notably, these authors excluded subjects with GFR <60 mL/min and 25-hydroxyvitamin D levels <30 ng/dL [12].

In a separate study, 6 of 100 postmenopausal women surveyed in Spain had NPHPT after excluding renal disease, vitamin D insufficiency (<30 pg/dL), and malnutrition [13].

In the Osteoporotic Fractures in Men (MrOS) population of men aged 65 years or older, the prevalence of NPHPT was 0.4 %. Separately, the Dallas Heart Study of men and women aged 18–65 years determined an initial prevalence of NPHPT of 3.1 %, a prevalence which decreased to 0.6 % after 8 years of follow-up, with some subjects having normalization of PTH levels, while others had progression to overt hypercalcemia [2].

The highest prevalence reported to date is 16.7 % as determined in the Canadian Multicentre Osteoporosis Study (CaMos) [14]. Of note, however, that study did not exclude patients with secondary hyperparathyroidism and used a lower limit of 25-hydroxyvitamin D levels of 20 ng/dL. Most recently, a survey of residents from a small village in Southern Italy found that 0.44 % of participants had NPHPT [15].

Gender predominance is also difficult to assess, as most cohorts studied to date have been gender specific. There does seem, however, to be a preponderance of NPHPT in the female gender [3, 16].

The histopathology of NPHPT follows other subgroups of PHPT: surgical resection has identified that most cases represent a single adenoma (80 %) followed by multiglandular hyperplasia (20 %) [11, 17]. A single case of carcinoma has been reported to date [18].

As noted previously, most studies that have evaluated subjects with NPHPT have included primarily referral populations, with most patients having symptoms related to their metabolic disease. Most notably, 25–57 % of subjects have osteoporosis on initial evaluation (either by bone mineral density (BMD) criteria or due to a history of fragility fractures), with 9–25 % having a history of nephrolithiasis [16, 17, 19–22].

In contrast to patients with asymptomatic mild PHPT in whom cortical bone loss occurs preferentially, osteoporosis in patients with NPHPT appears to be more common at the lumbar spine (34–66 %) and hip (38–47 %), with comparatively preserved bone mineral density at the distal one-third radius [16, 19, 23].

In a New York population-based cohort, up to 40 % of patients with NPHPT developed clinical features of PHPT including hypercalcemia, hypercalciuria, and/or significant bone loss during a median 3-year follow-up period [19, 22]. Patients who developed hypercalcemia on follow-up tended to be older and were more likely to have higher baseline values for serum calcium and urinary calcium [2, 19]. Such observations suggest the presence of an asymptomatic form of NPHPT that may only be identified in population-based screening. This is consistent with the dual-phase hypothesis proposed by Rao et al. in 1988 which suggested that the first biochemical abnormality of PHPT may be an elevated PTH level which is considered subclinical in the setting of a normal serum calcium value [24], a concept recently supported by Cusano et al. [2]. Hyperparathyroidism would thus be viewed as a spectrum that encompasses both normocalcemia and hypercalcemia and in parallel with, but not necessarily linked to, silent and symptomatic disease.

Several studies have evaluated cardiovascular disease and mortality in patients with hyperparathyroidism. In a number of these studies, PTH levels have been independently associated with increased incidence of cardiovascular disease irrespective of calcium levels. Indeed both hypercalcemic and normocalcemic subjects with elevated PTH levels had a higher prevalence of hypertension, with significantly elevated systolic and diastolic pressure measurements, when compared to subjects with normal PTH levels [25–27]. Other studies also found that in addition to hypertension, both hyperlipidemia and impaired fasting glucose are more prevalent in patients with hyperparathyroidism [28], along with an increased risk of death from cardiovascular causes [29].

Management

Recently, the Fourth International Workshop on the Management of Asymptomatic Primary Hyperparathyroidism identified the lack of substantial data permitting characterization of asymptomatic PHPT and its clinical and social impacts [30]. While NPHPT seems to have somewhat different clinical features than asymptomatic PHPT, both appear to represent a spectrum of the same disease. In the current absence of good evidence, management recommendations for asymptomatic PHPT may not be applicable to patients with NPHPT. Rather, an individualized approach to management is recommended.

Finally, the available literature that has examined changes in BMD after parathyroidectomy in patients with NPHPT demonstrated that 47 % of patients who underwent parathyroidectomy had preferential gains at the spine and hip as compared to the distal radius. A higher alkaline phosphatase activity presurgery was the best predictor of BMD improvement [23].

The aforementioned biochemical profile of the patient revealed mild hypercalciuria. Since idiopathic hypercalciuria could lead to secondary hyperparathyroidism, we elected to obtain a parathyroid scan looking for autonomous parathyroid function. The patient thus underwent ^{99m}Tc-sestamibi scintigraphy which demonstrated a discordant focus of activity posterior to the mid- to lower right thyroid lobe in the tracheoesophageal groove. This was consistent with a parathyroid adenoma.

Outcome

The presence of a parathyroid adenoma confirmed the presumed diagnosis of NPHPT. Given that the patient had a history of recurrent symptomatic nephrolithiasis and was at increased risk of recurrent nephrolithiasis given both hypercalciuria and hyperphosphaturia, she elected to proceed with surgical management due to her relatively young age and otherwise preserved general health.

Minimally invasive parathyroidectomy was performed with intraoperative serial PTH measurements (67.6 pg/mL at baseline and 26.8 pg/mL at 20 min). Pathology confirmed a 520-mg right superior parathyroid adenoma. Postoperative biochemical studies demonstrated serum calcium of 9.3 mg/dL, phosphorus of 3.8 mg/dL, and PTH of 30 pg/mL. When assessed 2 years postoperatively, the patient had not had recurrent nephrolithiasis.

Clinical Pearls/Pitfalls
- In contrast to PHPT patients in whom normal calcium levels may occur intermittently, patients with NPHPT are consistently normocalcemic on repeated evaluations.
- Excluding causes of secondary hyperparathyroidism is essential prior to making the diagnosis of NPHPT.
- NPHPT can remain silent for years; however, low bone mineral density and nephrolithiasis are common presenting features of the disease.
- PHPT is a spectrum that encompasses both normocalcemia and hypercalcemia that occurs in parallel with, but is not necessarily linked to, silent and symptomatic disease.
- While NPHPT seems to have somewhat different clinical features than asymptomatic PHPT, there currently is insufficient data to extrapolate management recommendations for asymptomatic PHPT to patients with NPHPT; an individualized approach to management is recommended.

Conflict of Interest   All authors state that they have no conflicts of interest.

References

1. Silverberg SJ, Bilezikian JP. "Incipient" primary hyperparathyroidism: a "Forme Fruste" of an old disease. J Clin Endocrinol Metab. 2003;88:5348–52.
2. Cusano NE, Maalouf NM, Wang PY, Zhang C, Cremers SC, Haney EM, et al. Normocalcemic hyperparathyroidism and hypoparathyroidism in two community-based nonreferral populations. J Clin Endocrinol Metab. 2013;98:2734–41.
3. Bilezikian JP, Silverberg SJ. Normocalcemic primary hyperparathyroidism. Arq Bras Endocrinol Metab. 2010;54:106–9.
4. Cusano NE, Silverberg SJ, Bilezikian JP. Normocalcemic primary hyperparathyroidism. J Clin Densitom. 2013;16:33–9.
5. Eastell R, Brandi ML, Costa AG, D'amour P, Shoback DM, Thakker RV. Diagnosis of asymptomatic primary hyperparathyroidism: Proceedings of the Fourth International Workshop. J Clin Endocrinol Metab. 2014;99(10):3570–9.
6. Ong GS, Walsh JP, Stuckey BG, et al. The importance of measuring ionized calcium in characterizing calcium status and diagnosing primary hyperparathyroidism. J Clin Endocrinol Metab. 2012;97:3138–45.
7. Björkman M, Sorva A, Tilvis R. Responses of parathyroid hormone to vitamin D supplementation: a systematic review of clinical trials. Arch Gerontol Geriatr. 2009;48:160–6.
8. Fillée C, Keller T, Mourad M, Brinkmann T, Ketelslegers JM. Impact of vitamin D-related serum PTH reference values on the diagnosis of mild primary hyperparathyroidism, using bivariate calcium/PTH reference regions. Clin Endocrinol (Oxf). 2012;76:785–9.
9. Kidney Disease: Improving Global Outcomes (KDIGO) CKD-MBD Work Group. KDIGO clinical practice guideline for the diagnosis, evaluation, prevention, and treatment of Chronic Kidney Disease-Mineral and Bone Disorder (CKD-MBD). Kidney Int Suppl. 2009;(113):S1–130.
10. National Kidney Foundation. K/DOQI clinical practice guidelines for bone metabolism and disease in chronic kidney disease. Am J Kidney Dis. 2003;42(4 Suppl 3):S1–201.
11. Lundgren E, Hagström EG, Lundin J, Winnerbäck K, Roos J, Ljunghall S, Rastad J. Primary hyperparathyroidism revisited in menopausal women with serum calcium in the upper normal range at population-based screening 8 years ago. World J Surg. 2002;26(8):931–6.
12. Misra B, Silverberg SJ, Bilezikian JP. Prevalence and demographics of asymptomatic normocalcemic hyperparathyroidism in the United

States. Program of the 30th Annual Meeting of the American Society of Bone and Mineral Research. Montreal; 2008.

13. Garcia-Martin A, Reyes-Garcia R, Munoz-Torres M. Normocalcemic primary hyperparathyroidism: one-year follow-up in one hundred post-menopausal women. Endocrine. 2012;42(3):764–6.

14. Berger C, Langsetmo L, Hanley D, Hadachi J, Kovacs C, Brown J, Josse R, Goltzman D. Relative prevalence of normocalcemic and hypercalcemic hyperparathyroidism in a community-dwelling cohort. 33rd Annual Meeting of the American Society of Bone and Mineral Research. San Diego; 2011. abstract pSU0173.

15. Vignali E, Cetani F, Chiavistelli S, Meola A, Saponaro F, Centoni R, et al. Normocalcemic primary hyperparathyroidism: a survey in a small village of Southern Italy. Endocr Connect. 2015;4(3):172–8.

16. Amaral LM, Queiroz DC, Marques TF, et al. Normocalcemic versus hypercalcemic primary hyperparathyroidism: more stone than bone? J Osteoporos. 2012;3:128–352.

17. Tordjman KM, Greenman Y, Osher E, et al. Characterization of normo-calcemic primary hyperparathyroidism. Am J Med. 2004;117:861–3.

18. Campennì A, Ruggeri RM, Sindoni A, Giovinazzo S, Calbo E, Ieni A, Calbo L, Tuccari G, Baldari S, Benvenga S. Parathyroid carcinoma presenting as normocalcemic hyperparathyroidism. J Bone Miner Metab. 2012;30:367–72.

19. Lowe H, McMahon DJ, Rubin MR, et al. Normocalcemic primary hyperparathyroidism: further characterization of a new clinical pheno-type. J Clin Endocrinol Metab. 2007;92:3001–5.

20. Cakir I, Unluhizarci K, Tanriverdi F, et al. Investigation of insulin resis-tance in patients with normocalcemic primary hyperparathyroidism. Endocrine. 2012;42(2):419–22.

21. Wade TJ, Yen TW, Amin AL, Wang TS. Surgical management of normo-calcemic primary hyperparathyroidism. World J Surg. 2012;36:761–6.

22. Liu J-M, Cusano NE, Silva BC, Zhao L, He X-Y, Tao B, et al. Primary hyperparathyroidism: a tale of two cities revisited – New York and Shanghai. Bone Res. 2013;2:162–9.

23. Koumakis E, Souberbielle J-C, Payet J, Sarfati E, Borderie D, Kahan A, et al. Individual site-specific bone mineral density gain in normocalce-mic primary hyperparathyroidism. Osteoporos Int. 2014;25:1963–8.

24. Rao DS, Wilson RJ, Kleerekoper M, Parfitt AM. Lack of biochemical progression or continuation of accelerated bone loss in mild asymptom-atic primary hyperparathyroidism: evidence for biphasic disease course. J Clin Endocrinol Metab. 1988;67(6):1294–8.

25. Yagi S, Aihara K, Kondo T, et al. High serum parathyroid hormone and calcium are risk factors for hypertension in Japanese patients. Endocr J. 2014;61:727–33.
26. Jorde R, Bonaa KH, Sundsfjord J. Population based study on serum ionised calcium, serum parathyroid hormone, and blood pressure. The Tromsø study. Eur J Endocrinol. 1999;141:350–7.
27. Chen G, Xue Y, Zhang Q, Xue T, Yao J, Huang H, et al. Is normocalcemic primary hyperparathyroidism: harmful or harmless? J Clin Endocrinol Metab. 2015;100(6):2420–4.
28. Tordjman KM, Yaron M, Izkhakov E, et al. Cardiovascular risk factors and arterial rigidity are similar in asymptomatic normocalcemic and hypercalcemic primary hyperparathyroidism. Eur J Endocrinol. 2010; 162:925–33.
29. Hedbäck G, Odén A. Increased risk of death from primary hyperparathyroidism – an update. Eur J Clin Invest. 1998;28:271–6.
30. Silverberg SJ, Clarke BL, Peacock M, Bandeira F, Boutroy S, Cusano NE, et al. Current issues in the presentation of asymptomatic primary hyperparathyroidism: Proceedings of the Fourth International Workshop. J Clin Endocrinol Metab. 2014;99(10):3580–94.

Chapter 19
Secondary Hyperparathyroidism

Nishanth Vallumsetla, Manpreet S. Mundi,
and Kurt A. Kennel

Case Presentation

A 46-year-old woman was referred for evaluation of low bone
mineral density (BMD) detected during evaluation for surgical
management of lumbar radiculopathy. She had never experienced
a fracture and routine lumbar and thoracic spine films showed no
vertebral deformities. Other than radicular pain in her right lower
extremity treated with gabapentin, she felt well and was without
complaint on review of systems. Her prior medical history was
notable for depression treated with fluoxetine, Roux-en-Y gastric
bypass for the treatment of obesity 6 years prior, and amenorrhea
following endometrial ablation. To date she had not experienced
menopausal symptoms. In the past year, she denies use of other
prescription or over-the-counter medications or supplements. She
had never smoked and abstains from consuming alcohol. She had
limited knowledge of her family's medical history.

N. Vallumsetla, MBBS • M.S. Mundi, MD • K.A. Kennel, MD (✉)
Division of Endocrinology, Diabetes, Metabolism, and Nutrition,
Department of Internal Medicine, Mayo College of Medicine,
Mayo Clinic, Rochester, MN, USA
e-mail: vallumsetla.nishanth@mayo.edu; mundi.manpreet@mayo.edu;
kennel.kurt@mayo.edu

A.E. Kearns, R.A. Wermers (eds.), *Hyperparathyroidism:*
A Clinical Casebook, DOI 10.1007/978-3-319-25880-5_19,
© Mayo Foundation for Medical Education and Research 2016

An evaluation for secondary causes of low BMD included laboratory assessment which revealed serum calcium 9.0 mg/dL (nl, 8.9–10.1), phosphorus 2.5 mg/dL (nl, 2.5–4.5), albumin 4.4 g/dL (nl, 3.5–5.0), serum creatinine 0.8 mg/dL (nl, 0.6–1.0), 25-OH vitamin D 35 ng/mL (nl, 20–50), and total alkaline phosphatase 111 U/L (nl, 39–100) with otherwise normal liver function tests. Follicle-stimulating hormone was within the premenopausal reference range. In part due to her surgeon's request for consideration of preoperative teriparatide (rPTH 1–34) therapy, serum parathyroid hormone (PTH) was measured and retuned elevated at 194 pg/mL (nl, 15–65).

Assessment and Diagnosis

An elevation in PTH in the presence of hypercalcemia indicates PTH-mediated hypercalcemia [1]. In contrast, several mechanisms and diagnoses must be entertained when PTH elevations are associated with normal serum calcium concentrations. Even so, initially characterizing the elevation of PTH as secondary rather than primary is important as a working diagnosis of secondary hyperparathyroidism (SHP) simultaneously leads to a search for causes and options for treatment that have the potential to normalize PTH. Misdiagnosis of primary hyperparathyroidism may lead to misleading localization studies and unnecessary surgery [2]. Given disorders leading to secondary hyperparathyroidism often have broad implications for health, pursuing the cause(s) of SHP aims to accomplish more for the patient than just normalizing PTH. Occasionally, but always subsequent to a vigorous evaluation for secondary causes of hyperparathyroidism, normocalcemic primary hyperparathyroidism may be added to the differential diagnosis (see Chap. 18) [3]. The mechanism of disorders of calcium or phosphorus homeostasis leading to secondary hyperparathyroidism can be loosely divided as follows: inadequate nutrition, malabsorption, altered excretion, altered mobilization, and impaired PTH action.

Extracellular ionized calcium (iCa) is tightly regulated by PTH in response to signaling through the calcium sensing receptor (CaSR) on the parathyroid glands. A decline in iCa below an individual's set point triggers release of PTH, which has a three-pronged action to restore calcium levels. Most immediate is increased reabsorption of calcium from the glomerular filtrate. If relative hypocalcemia persists, PTH activates enzymatic conversion of 25-hydroxyvitamin D to 1,25-dihydroxyvitamin D (calcitriol) in the kidneys. Calcitriol in turn augments calcium uptake from the gut through increased active transport across the small intestinal mucosa. If necessary to address a continuing calcium deficit, PTH mobilizes calcium from the skeleton released through activation of osteoclastic bone resorption via its effects on RANK ligand (RANKL) and osteoprotegerin [4].

Given obligatory losses of calcium through sweat, urine, and feces, calcium balance requires a sufficient daily dietary intake. The recommended daily allowance (RDA) of calcium is calculated based on obligatory daily losses of calcium and an estimated rate of absorption of calcium from diet. For PTH to indirectly improve calcium absorption, sufficient vitamin D as a substrate for calcitriol production is essential. The RDA of vitamin D for the prevention of overt skeletal disease is 600–800 IU depending in part on age [5]. A survey of foods consumed by this patient made evident that her intake of dairy, other calcium-rich foods, and foods providing vitamin D were well below suggested intakes. Although micronutrient supplementation has the potential to bridge the gap in those whose diets are insufficient, this patient reported poor adherence to the micronutrient supplementation she had previously been recommended to consume. Cutaneous production of vitamin D in response to sunlight exposure is highly variable yet can be the dominant source of vitamin D in many individuals [6]. That her 25 hydroxyvitamin D concentration was normal attests to the effectiveness of passive sun exposure during the summer when she presented.

The majority of calcium absorption occurs by passive paracellular absorption [7]. Although vitamin D-dependent absorption is important especially when dietary calcium intake is low, vitamin D sufficiency does not exclude calcium malabsorption as a cause for secondary hyperparathyroidism. In malabsorption syndromes (celiac disease, Crohn's disease, cholestatic liver disease, bariatric surgery, short bowel, etc.), poor absorption or decreased intestinal length may compromise the availability of dietary-derived vitamin D and calcium leading to negative calcium balance and PTH release. This patient had undergone bariatric surgery which commonly is associated with secondary hyperparathyroidism [8–11]. In addition to restricting the breadth of her diet and quantity of nutrients consumed, a gastric bypass reduces the fractional absorption of calcium [12, 13], thus compounding her dietary deficit.

Assessing renal excretion of calcium provides indirect evidence of insufficiency of dietary calcium intake, calcium malabsorption, and/or vitamin D deficiency leading to SHP. The majority of calcium reabsorption from the glomerular filtrate occurs in the proximal tubule independent of PTH [14]. Still, a considerable amount of calcium reabsorption is controlled at the cortical thick ascending limb of loop of Henle (via PTH and independent function of CaSR) and the distal convoluted tubule (via PTH) [15, 16]. Although the reference range for urinary excretion of calcium in normal adults is wide, ranging between 40 and 250 mg per 24 h period, values less than 100 mg in the setting of vitamin D sufficiency raise suspicion for insufficiency of dietary calcium intake or calcium malabsorption especially when accompanied by PTH elevation. Consistent with her dietary and surgical history, this patient's 24 h urine calcium was 54 mg per spec on a complete collection as confirmed by creatinine measurement.

Hyperphosphatemia largely occurs in the context of kidney disease. In the absence of advanced chronic kidney disease, the need to measure serum phosphorus may be overlooked when evaluating elevated PTH. Phosphate can bind to iCa leading to increased production of PTH. Hyperphosphatemia also causes increased production of FGF23 which inhibits conversion of vitamin D to calcitriol [17]. Serum phosphorus also has direct stimulatory effects on PTH production [18]. Transient and severe hyperphosphatemia can occur due to oral supplements or enemas, massive tissue injury, or tumor lysis. Chronic hyperphosphatemia which commonly occurs in chronic kidney disease, in conjunction with decreased activation of vitamin D to calcitriol, is a common cause of SHP and parathyroid hyperplasia [17]. In cases of unexplained secondary hyperparathyroidism, if the degree to which renal function (typically GFR <50 mL/min) and 1-alpha hydroxylase activity are impaired is unclear, measurement of 1,25-dihydroxyvitamin D concentration may be considered. This patient had normal renal function as evidenced by a normal serum creatinine concentration. Her serum phosphorus concentration was at the lower end of the reference range consistent with the phosphaturic effects of PTH at the proximal tubule [19].

If a calcium deficit is chronic, leading to chronic PTH-mediated bone resorption, biochemical markers of bone turnover may rise within the reference range or be frankly elevated. The development of osteomalacia may be evident by fracture, bone pain, overt hypocalcemia, and/or hypophosphatemia yet takes years of persistent calcium and/or phosphorus deficits to occur. In this patient, total serum alkaline phosphatase was elevated without other evidence of liver disease. Subsequent direct measurement of bone specific alkaline phosphatase was 23 mcg/L (nl, <14 in premenopausal women). Although unproven without histologic examination of bone tissue, this patient's low BMD may reflect bone demineralization. In such settings, treatment of underlying conditions, restoration of normal calcium and phosphorus homeostasis, and resolution of secondary hyperparathyroidism can result in significant improvement in BMD [20]. As such, pharmacotherapy to increase BMD should initially be deferred.

Although undesirable, mobilization of the skeletal mineral is a necessary component of the compensatory effect of PTH to minimize the decline in serum calcium concentrations. Antiresorptive therapy in this setting will markedly attenuate the efflux of calcium and may precipitate overt and symptomatic hypocalcemia [21]. Even in patients with normal calcium homeostasis, potent antiresorptive therapy for metabolic bone disease (e.g., osteoporosis) or cancer causes a transient decline in serum iCa and rise in PTH for several weeks [22]. Patients with high bone turnover (thus increased flux of calcium into and out of bone) due to other metabolic bone disease (e.g., Paget's disease) may also display a rise in PTH with potent antiresorptive therapy [23, 24].

When factors related to nutrition, absorption, mobilization, and excretion of calcium, phosphorus, and vitamin D are excluded, disorders of impaired PTH action should be considered. Magnesium (Mg) depletion may occur in conjunction with calcium malabsorption. Although chronic hypomagnesemia, such as that associated with proton pump inhibitor therapy, is most often associated with functional hypoparathyroidism, acute hypomagnesemia can cause functional PTH resistance [25]. Heritable PTH resistance syndromes such as pseudohypoparathyroidism may be suspected based on physical features, other hormonal resistance, or timing of onset.

Management

Aided by a registered dietitian nutritionist, the patient increased her dietary intake of low-fat dairy products. Concurrently she reinstituted routine postgastric bypass micronutrient supplementation daily multivitamin with minerals, monthly cyanocobalamin injection, and two calcium citrate 315 mg tablets with her midday and evening meal [26, 27]. She was given a goal of 1600–2000 mg total calcium intake per day. After discussion with the patient and her surgeon, surgery was deferred so long as her radiculopathy was not evolving to include muscle weakness or related functional impairment.

Outcome

Reassessment 3 months later showed serum calcium 9.4 mg/dL (nl, 8.9–10.1), phosphorus 3.2 mg/dL (nl, 2.5–4.5), PTH 33 pg/ mL (nl, 15–65), total alkaline phosphatase 89 U/L (nl, 39–100), and 24 h urine calcium 124 mg per spec (desired postgastric bypass in our practice >100 mg). She then underwent laminectomy and L4–L5 fusion with an uneventful recovery. As she was premenopausal, had not experienced fragility fractures, and may see an improvement in her BMD with correction of her nutritional deficiency, pharmacotherapy to improve bone strength was deferred. She was recommended to have repeat BMD assessment in 1 year and/or at the onset of symptoms of menopause.

Clinical Pearls/Pitfalls
- In patients with normal serum calcium and phosphorus, a vigorous assessment for potential causes for physiologic (i.e., secondary) PTH elevations is essential before considering disorders characterized by autonomous production of PTH.
- Avoid performing localization studies as a primary step in evaluating elevations in PTH that may not be due to primary hyperparathyroidism.

- SHP in the presence of normal serum calcium, serum phosphorus, vitamin D stores, and renal function may represent compensation (i.e., the serum calcium is maintained in the reference range) for primary calcium insufficiency or malabsorption.
- When suspected, assessing renal excretion of calcium can provide indirect evidence of insufficiency of dietary calcium intake or calcium malabsorption leading to SHP.
- Treatment of factors suspected of causing SHP is both diagnostic and therapeutic.
- Longstanding SHP leading to parathyroid hyperplasia may take longer to resolve.

Conflict of Interest   All authors state that they have no conflicts of interest.

References

1. Eastell R, Brandi ML, Costa AG, D'Amour P, Shoback DM, Thakker RV. Diagnosis of asymptomatic primary hyperparathyroidism: proceedings of the Fourth International Workshop. J Clin Endocrinol Metab. 2014;99(10):3570–9.
2. Kirkby-Bott J, El-Khatib Z, Soudan B, Caiazzo R, Arnalsteen L, Carnaille B. 25-hydroxy vitamin D deficiency causes parathyroid incidentalomas. Langenbecks Arch Surg. 2010;395(7):919–24.
3. Cusano NE, Silverberg SJ, Bilezikian JP. Normocalcemic primary hyperparathyroidism. J Clin Densitom. 2013;16(1):33–9.
4. Xiong J, Piemontese M, Thostenson JD, Weinstein RS, Manolagas SC, O'Brien CA. Osteocyte-derived RANKL is a critical mediator of the increased bone resorption caused by dietary calcium deficiency. Bone. 2014;66:146–54.
5. Ross AC, Manson JE, Abrams SA, Aloia JF, Brannon PM, Clinton SK, et al; Institute of Medicine. Dietary reference intakes for calcium and vitamin D. Washington, DC: The National Academies Press; 2011.

6. Lips P, van Schoor NM, de Jongh RT. Diet, sun, and lifestyle as determinants of vitamin D status. Ann N Y Acad Sci. 2014;1317:92–8.
7. Hoenderop JGJ, Nilius B, Bindels RJM. Calcium absorption across epithelia. Physiol Rev. 2004;85(1):373–422.
8. Lozano O, García-Díaz JD, Cancer E, Arribas I, Rubio JL, González-García I, et al. Phosphocalcic metabolism after biliopancreatic diversion. Obes Surg. 2007;17(5):642–8.
9. Moizé V, Andreu A, Flores L, Torres F, Ibarzabal A, Delgado S, et al. Long-term dietary intake and nutritional deficiencies following sleeve gastrectomy or Roux-En-Y gastric bypass in a Mediterranean population. J Acad Nutr Diet. 2013;113(3):400–10.
10. Moreiro J, Ruiz O, Perez G, Salinas R, Urgeles JR, Riesco M, et al. Parathyroid hormone and bone marker levels in patients with morbid obesity before and after biliopancreatic diversion. Obes Surg. 2007;17(3):348–54.
11. Valderas JP, Velasco S, Solari S, Liberona Y, Viviani P, Maiz A, et al. Increase of bone resorption and the parathyroid hormone in postmenopausal women in the long-term after Roux-en-Y gastric bypass. Obes Surg. 2009;19(8):1132–8.
12. Riedt CS, Brolin RE, Sherrell RM, Field MP, Shapses SA. True fractional calcium absorption is decreased after Roux-En-Y gastric bypass surgery. Obesity. 2006;14(11):1940–8.
13. Schafer AL, Weaver CM, Black DM, Wheeler AL, Chang H, Szefc GV, et al. Intestinal calcium absorption decreases dramatically after gastric bypass surgery despite optimization of vitamin D status. J Bone Miner Res. 2015;30(8):1377–85.
14. Nordin B, Peacock M. Role of kidney in regulation of plasma-calcium. Lancet. 1969;294(7633):1280–3.
15. Riccardi D, Hall AE, Chattopadhyay N, Xu JZ, Brown EM, Hebert SC. Localization of the extracellular Ca2+/polyvalent cation-sensing protein in rat kidney. Am J Physiol Ren Physiol. 1998;274(3):F611–22.
16. de Groot T, Lee K, Langeslag M, Xi Q, Jalink K, Bindels RJ, et al. Parathyroid hormone activates TRPV5 via PKA-dependent phosphorylation. J Am Soc Nephrol. 2009;20(8):1693–704.
17. Goodman WG, Quarles LD. Development and progression of secondary hyperparathyroidism in chronic kidney disease: lessons from molecular genetics. Kidney Int. 2007;74(3):276–88.
18. Kilav R, Silver J, Naveh-Many T. Parathyroid hormone gene expression in hypophosphatemic rats. J Clin Investig. 1995;96(1):327–33.
19. Pfister MF, Lederer E, Forgo J, Ziegler U, Lötscher M, Quabius ES, et al. Parathyroid hormone-dependent degradation of type II Na+/Pi cotransporters. J Biol Chem. 1997;272(32):20125–30.

20. Basha B, Rao DS, Han Z-H, Parfitt AM. Osteomalacia due to vitamin D depletion: a neglected consequence of intestinal malabsorption. Am J Med. 2000;108(4):296–300.
21. Rosen CJ, Brown S. Severe hypocalcemia after intravenous bisphosphonate therapy in occult vitamin D deficiency. N Engl J Med. 2003; 348(15):1503–4.
22. Dicuonzo G, Vincenzi B, Santini D, Avvisati G, Rocci L, Battistoni F, et al. Fever after zoledronic acid administration is due to increase in TNF-α and IL-6. J Interferon Cytokine Res. 2003;23(11):649–54.
23. Qi W-X, Lin F, He A-N, Tang L-N, Shen Z, Yao Y. Incidence and risk of denosumab-related hypocalcemia in cancer patients: a systematic review and pooled analysis of randomized controlled studies. Curr Med Res Opin. 2013;29(9):1067–73.
24. Kreutle V, Blum C, Meier C, Past M, Muller B, Schutz P, et al. Bisphosphonate induced hypocalcaemia – report of six cases and review of the literature. Swiss Med Wkly. 2014;144:w13979.
25. Yamamoto M, Yamaguchi T, Yamauchi M, Yano S, Sugimoto T. Acute-onset hypomagnesemia-induced hypocalcemia caused by the refractoriness of bones and renal tubules to parathyroid hormone. J Bone Miner Metab. 2011;29(6):752–5.
26. Mechanick JI, Kushner RF, Sugerman HJ, Gonzalez-Campoy JM, Collazo-Clavell ML, Spitz AF, et al. American Association of Clinical Endocrinologists, the Obesity Society, and American Society for Metabolic & Bariatric Surgery medical guidelines for clinical practice for the perioperative nutritional, metabolic, and nonsurgical support of the bariatric surgery patient. Obesity. 2009;17(S1):S3–72.
27. Tondapu P, Provost D, Adams-Huet B, Sims T, Chang C, Sakhaee K. Comparison of the absorption of calcium carbonate and calcium citrate after Roux-en-Y gastric bypass. Obes Surg. 2009;19(9):1256–61.

Chapter 20
Tertiary Hyperparathyroidism

Kurt A. Kennel and Bart L. Clarke

Case Presentation

A 47-year-old female initially presented at age 13 with intermittent paresthesias and tetany associated with hypocalcemia (5.5 mg/dL, normal, 9.5–10.4), hyperphosphatemia (8.4 mg/dL, normal, 4.0–5.2), increased parathyroid hormone (PTH) (8.5 pmol/L, normal, 1.0–5.2), and mild osteitis fibrosa on bone biopsy. She had no features of Albright's hereditary osteodystrophy or family history of hypocalcemia. She was treated with calcium and vitamin D supplementation and her symptoms resolved. Repeat bone biopsy showed healed osteitis fibrosa. Subsequently, her urine cyclic AMP (cAMP) was found unresponsive to exogenous PTH, and she was diagnosed with pseudohypoparathyroidism (PHP) type Ib. During the ensuing years, she reported intermittent paresthesias associated with mild

K.A. Kennel, MD (✉) • B.L. Clarke, MD
Division of Endocrinology, Diabetes, Metabolism, and Nutrition,
Department of Internal Medicine, Mayo College of Medicine,
Mayo Clinic, Rochester, MN, USA
e-mail: kennel.kurt@mayo.edu; clarke.bart@mayo.edu

A.E. Kearns, R.A. Wermers (eds.), *Hyperparathyroidism:*
A Clinical Casebook, DOI 10.1007/978-3-319-25880-5_20,
© Mayo Foundation for Medical Education and Research 2016

hypocalcemia on supplemental elemental calcium of 1800 mg, 1,25-dihydroxyvitamin D (calcitriol) 0.25 mcg, and hydrochlorothiazide 25 mg each day.

In the year prior to her current presentation, her serum PTH concentrations increased dramatically above her baseline level, and her serum calcium became mildly elevated despite lack of changes in her medications and diet or due to other medical conditions. At her initial evaluation, she was asymptomatic and had in fact not experienced paresthesias for quite some time. Her overall health was excellent, with no history of fractures or kidney stones. Other than relatively short stature (155 cm), her physical examination was unremarkable, including a normal thyroid examination. Her initial laboratory assessment included serum calcium 10.2 mg/dL (normal, 8.9–10.1), phosphorus 3.2 mg/dL (normal, 2.5–4.5), creatinine 0.9 g/dL (normal, 0.6–0.9), and PTH 21 pmol/L (normal, 1.0–5.2).

Assessment and Diagnosis

The primary function of the parathyroid glands is to secrete PTH in response to a fall in the blood ionized calcium (iCa) concentration as "measured" by the calcium-sensing receptor (CaSR) on the plasma membrane [1, 2]. Short-term and modest decreases in iCa result in the release of stored PTH from secretory vesicles, decreased intracellular degradation of PTH stores, and increased PTH mRNA expression and lifespan. This physiologic or secondary hyperparathyroidism (SHP) may normalize iCa by increasing renal reabsorption of iCa, by increasing intestinal absorption of iCa by increasing renal production of 1,25 dihydroxyvitamin D, and by increasing osteoclastic activity and mobilization of calcium from the skeleton. However, should dietary calcium intake or absorption be limited, 25 hydroxyvitamin D be deficient, and bone mineral be depleted, overt and chronically low iCa may occur, stimulating an increase in the number of PTH-secreting parathyroid cells (i.e., hyperplasia) and the potential for even higher serum PTH concentrations [3].

Parathyroid gland function and growth is also regulated by plasma phosphate and 1,25 dihydroxyvitamin D concentrations. In chronic kidney disease (CKD), increased binding of plasma phosphate to ionized calcium in the setting of hyperphosphatemia and reduced intestinal calcium absorption due to inadequate production of 1,25 dihydroxyvitamin D can both contribute to a decline in iCa. Increases in FGF-23 that suppress 1,25-dihydroxyvitamin D production and decrease vitamin D receptors in parathyroid tissue in advanced CKD both reduce suppression of PTH secretion [4]. Simultaneously, increasing serum phosphate concentrations have a direct effect on parathyroid glands resulting in increased PTH synthesis and by promoting the stability of PTH mRNA [5]. Ultimately, any disorder that persistently disturbs multiple targets of or modifiers of PTH action leading to hypocalcemia and/or hyperphosphatemia can greatly stimulate parathyroid gland function and growth through multiple clinically modifiable mechanisms.

Although most commonly associated with CKD, malabsorption, and vitamin D deficiency, SHP also occurs due to failure of target tissues to respond to the actions of PTH. PTH resistance occurs in the proximal renal tubule as evidenced by lack of phosphaturic response and increased cAMP excretion with exogenous PTH administration as was seen in the case above [6]. In other target tissues, PTH action remains intact including in the thick ascending tubule which likely explains relative hypocalciuria compared to patients with hypoparathyroidism [7]. That PTH action remains in bone [8] has been demonstrated clinically [9, 10] and histologically in the case above at first presentation with osteitis fibrosa. Similar to other causes of SHP, treatment of PHP includes calcium supplementation, phosphate restriction, and calcitriol treatment intended to normalize serum calcium and phosphorus which in turn will reduce multiple stimuli of PTH production and parathyroid gland growth.

Tertiary hyperparathyroidism (THP) is characterized by excessive secretion of PTH after long-standing SHP, and which may now include hypercalcemia [11]. THP can be the end result of long-standing SHP in which the parathyroid glands now exhibit autonomous function even after correction of underlying disease (e.g., post renal transplantation) [12]. The cellular etiology of THP is unknown but is postulated to be a result of a monoclonal expansion of parathyroid cells [13]. It is believed that these cells have an altered set point of their calcium-sensing receptor (CaSR) so that PTH is secreted despite elevated iCa concentrations [14].

Patients with long-standing chronic stimulation of their parathyroid glands often develop autonomy, such that they do not respond to calcium and calcitriol supplementation or phosphate restriction in their diet. In this situation, little can be done to stop overproduction of PTH short of parathyroidectomy, although certain interventions may be successful in temporarily reducing excess secretion of parathyroid hormone. Phosphate binders such as calcium acetate, sevelamer, or lanthanum are usually used to control hyperphosphatemia in patients where dietary restriction of phosphorus to 800–1000 mg each day is not sufficient. Lowering serum phosphorus may help lower FGF-23 and PTH secretion also as described above.

Certain synthetic active vitamin D analogues such as paricalcitol, doxercalciferol, and others have been shown to reduce PTH secretion by moderate amounts without simultaneously stimulating absorption of calcium and phosphate by the intestine. These have a modulating effect on the amount of PTH release by autonomous glands by direct transcriptional inhibition of PTH synthesis in the parathyroid glands and tend to reduce circulating PTH concentrations [15, 16]. Higher doses of these agents may lead to an increase in serum calcium or phosphate by stimulating intestinal absorption and tend to increase FGF-23 levels.

Cinacalcet is a calcimimetic compound that effectively lowers PTH secretion by autonomous or semiautonomous parathyroid glands. This allosteric sensitizer of the calcium-sensing receptor causes parathyroid chief cells to sense higher levels of extracellular calcium than are actually present, leading to decreased production of PTH, which leads to decreased serum calcium [17–19]. Cinacalcet is typically started at 30 mg once daily, with follow-up serum calcium measurement within 1 week. The most common side effect is nausea with vomiting, but taking cinacalcet with meals minimizes these side effects. Hypocalcemia may also occur, and cinacalcet should not be given if serum calcium is less than 8.4 mg/dL. Cinacalcet may be titrated upward to a maximum of 90 mg four times daily in the setting of parathyroid cancer, but is titrated to a maximum of 60 mg three times daily for THP. Patients with THP are usually at least moderately responsive to cinacalcet.

Hemodialysis or peritoneal dialysis will help control calcium and phosphorus abnormalities in end-stage chronic kidney disease, but usually do not help reduce PTH secretion in most patients. Renal transplantation corrects many abnormalities as long as the transplanted kidney continues to function well, and usually helps improve PTH secretion overall, but not in all cases.

For patients who have persistent THP despite optimal medical management, or after beginning dialysis treatment, or undergoing renal transplantation, surgery is usually recommended as a last resort. Because patients with THP typically have all four parathyroid glands oversecreting PTH, surgery usually removes three and one-half glands or all four glands with autotransplantation of a part of one gland into the neck, chest, or forearm muscle. Surgery to remove three and one-half glands leaves the remaining half-gland in place with intact blood supply. Autotransplantation of one-half gland usually leads to revascularization of the parathyroid tissue from surrounding muscle blood supply. In both cases, success of control of PTH oversecretion is high, and risk of hypoparathyroidism is low. In some cases four-gland hyperplasia is associated with four mildly to moderately enlarged glands of the about same size, but in other cases, asymmetry is noted, with some glands larger than the others. In patients who develop recurrent THP later due to continued autonomy of the half-gland left in situ or autotransplanted, medical therapy may be tried again, and if this fails, surgery may be recommended again. Repeat surgery for THP is associated with a higher risk of hypoparathyroidism [20].

In the case presented, it is presumed that suboptimal calcium or calcitriol replacement led to chronic mild hypocalcemia, which led to chronic stimulation of her parathyroid glands. At some point one or more of her parathyroid glands became autonomously secreting, and she developed THP with hypercalcemia. Cessation of her paresthesias was a harbinger of development of THP.

Management

Bone mineral density for the case discussed was above average for age and gender (T-score = 1.2, Z-score = 3.1). Parathyroid sestamibi scan and neck ultrasound each suggested two enlarged inferior parathyroid glands. At surgery, both the right and left inferior parathyroid glands were visibly enlarged, whereas the superior glands were of normal size and appearance. Baseline intraoperative PTH was 43.7 pmol/L. After the right inferior 720-mg gland was removed, PTH decreased to 31 pmol/L. After the left inferior 130-mg gland was removed, PTH decreased further to 6.9 pmol/L (Fig. 20.1). Histopathology indicated parathyroid hyperplasia in both glands. Tissue tumor markers Ki-67 and p27 were normal, thus not suggestive of malignant transformation. Postoperative serum calcium decreased to 8.6 mg/dL, with a PTH nadir of 3.3 pmol/L. Remaining asymptomatic, she began oral calcium supplementation of 2400 mg and 1,25-dihydroxyvitamin D 0.50 mcg daily. By postoperative day three serum calcium was normal at 9.2 mg/dL. Two weeks later, serum calcium remained normal and PTH had increased to

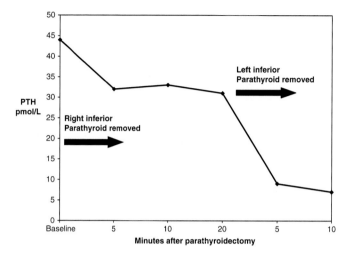

Fig. 20.1 Intraoperative parathyroid hormone levels after sequential resection of hyperplastic right inferior and left inferior parathyroid glands to treat tertiary hyperparathyroidism in a patient with pseudohypoparathyroidism type Ib

16.3 pmol/L (1.3–7.6), indicating return of function of remaining parathyroid tissue and suggesting mild residual hyperparathyroidism in her remaining glands.

Outcome

At 10-year follow-up, she felt well. Her serum calcium remained in the normal range with consistent use of 1000 mg elemental calcium daily, 1,25-dihydroxyvitamin D 0.25 mcg daily, and hydrochlorothiazide 25 mg every other day over 10 years of follow-up. PTH remained elevated but stable at 7.8 pmol/L. BMD remained normal and above average for age.

Clinical Pearls/Pitfalls

- Chronic stimulation by mild ionized hypocalcemia due to chronic PTH resistance and related disorders may result in parathyroid gland hyperplasia and even greater extent of PTH elevation sufficient to cause mild hypercalcemia.
- Tissue-specific decreases in Gsα expression in the proximal renal tubules with preserved expression in bone and other tissues may be clinically evident in disorders such as pseudohypoparathyroidism type Ib and may influence determination of optimal PTH concentrations in such patients.
- In patients with underlying conditions for whom elevated serum concentrations of PTH may be necessary to optimize physiologic functions related to calcium and phosphorus, need for and extent of parathyroidectomy should be carefully discussed with an endocrine surgeon.

Conflicts of Interest All authors state that they have no conflicts of interest.

References

1. Brown EM, Gamba G, Riccardi D, Lombardi M, Butters R, Kifor O, et al. Cloning and characterization of an extracellular Ca2+-sensing receptor from bovine parathyroid. Nature. 1993;366(6455):575–80.
2. Grant F, Conlin P, Brown E. Rate and concentration dependence of parathyroid hormone dynamics during stepwise changes in serum ionized calcium in normal humans. J Clin Endocrinol Metab. 1990; 71:370–8.
3. Jüppner H, Gardella T, Brown E. Parathyroid hormone and parathyroid hormone-related peptide in the regulation of calcium homeostasis and bone development. In: DeGroot L, Jameson J, editors. Endocrinology: adult and pediatric. 7th ed. Philadelphia: Elsevier; 2015.

4. Goodman WG, Quarles LD. Development and progression of secondary hyperparathyroidism in chronic kidney disease: lessons from molecular genetics. Kidney Int. 2007;74:276–88.
5. Moallem E, Kilav R, Silver J, Naveh-Many T. RNA-protein binding and post-transcriptional regulation of parathyroid hormone gene expression by calcium and phosphate. J Biol Chem. 1998;273:5253–9.
6. Mallette LE. Synthetic human parathyroid hormone 1-34 fragment for diagnostic testing. Ann Intern Med. 1988;109:800–4.
7. Stone MD, Hosking DJ, Garcia-Himmelstine C, White DA, Rosenblum D, Worth HG. The renal response to exogenous parathyroid hormone in treated pseudohypoparathyroidism. Bone. 1993;14:727–35.
8. Ish-Shalom S, Rao LG, Levine MA, Fraser D, Kooh SW, Josse RG, et al. Normal parathyroid hormone responsiveness of bone-derived cells from a patient with pseudohypoparathyroidism. J Bone Miner Res. 1996;11:8–14.
9. Zvi F. Pseudohypohyperparathyroidism-pseudohypoparathyroidism type Ib. J Bone Miner Res. 1999;14:1016.
10. Tollin SR, Perlmutter S, Aloia JF. Serial changes in bone mineral density and bone turnover after correction of secondary hyperparathyroidism in a patient with pseudohypoparathyroidism type Ib. J Bone Miner Res. 2000;15:1412–6.
11. Park-Sigal J, Don BR, Porzig A, Recker R, Griswold V, Sebastian A, et al. Severe hypercalcemic hyperparathyroidism developing in a patient with hyperaldosteronism and renal resistance to parathyroid hormone. J Bone Miner Res. 2013;28:700–8.
12. Bleskestad IH, Bergrem H, Leivestad T, Gøransson LG. Intact parathyroid hormone levels in renal transplant patients with normal transplant function. Clin Transplant. 2011;25:E566–70.
13. Krause MW, Hedinger CE. Pathologic study of parathyroid glands in tertiary hyperparathyroidism. Hum Pathol. 1985;16:772–84.
14. Grzela T, Chudzinski W, Lasiecka Z, Niderla J, Wilczynski G, Gornicka B, et al. The calcium-sensing receptor and vitamin D receptor expression in tertiary hyperparathyroidism. Int J Mol Med. 2006;17:779–83.
15. Palmer SC, McGregor DO, Macaskill P, Craig JC, Elder GJ, Strippoli GFM. Meta-analysis: vitamin D compounds in chronic kidney disease. Ann Intern Med. 2007;147:840–53.
16. Zisman AL, Ghantous W, Schinleber P, Roberts L, Sprague SM. Inhibition of parathyroid hormone: a dose equivalency study of paricalcitol and doxercalciferol. Am J Nephrol. 2005;25:591–5.
17. Indridason OS, Quarles LD. Comparison of treatments for mild secondary hyperparathyroidism in hemodialysis patients. Kidney Int. 2000;57:282–92.

18. Lindberg JS, Moe SM, Goodman WG, Coburn JW, Sprague SM, Liu W, et al. The calcimimetic AMG 073 reduces parathyroid hormone and calcium x phosphorus in secondary hyperparathyroidism. Kidney Int. 2003;63:248–54.
19. Koizumi M, Komaba H, Nakanishi S, Fujimori A, Fukagawa M. Cinacalcet treatment and serum FGF23 levels in haemodialysis patients with secondary hyperparathyroidism. Nephrol Dial Transplant. 2012;27:784–90.
20. Pitt SC, Sippel RS, Chen H. Secondary and tertiary hyperparathyroid-ism, state of the art surgical management. Surg Clin North Am. 2009;89:1227–39.

Index

A.E. Kearns, R.A. Wermers (eds.), *Hyperparathyroidism: A Clinical Casebook*, DOI 10.1007/978-3-319-25880-5
© Mayo Foundation for Medical Education and Research 2016

PTH. *See* Parathyroid hormone
    (PTH)
PTHrP. *See* Parathyroid hormone-
    related peptide (PTHrP)
Purified protein derivative (PPD)
    skin testing, 142

Q
Quantiferon measurement, 142

R
Radiation, for parathyroid
    carcinoma, 92
Raloxifene
    for bone mineral density,
        112, 113
    and serum calcium levels, 151
Recommended daily allowance
    (RDA), 171
Renal excretion, and SHP, 172
Renal stone disease, 123
Renal transplantation, 183
Renin-angiotensin-aldosterone
    system inhibitors, and
    PTH secretion, 152
Rheumatoid factor, 42
rhPTH. *See* Teriparatide (rhPTH)
Risedronate, for bone mineral
    density, 38, 112, 113

S
Sandwich-type immunometric
    assays, 39
Sarcoidosis, 142, 144, 145
Secondary hyperparathyroidism
    (SHP), 169–176, 182.
    See also Tertiary
    hyperparathyroidism
    (TPH)

causes of, 162
Selective venous sampling
    (SVS), 61
Serial sample dilutions, 39–40
Serum creatinine, and
    asymptomatic PHPT, 4
Sestamibi scan, 30, 34,
    49, 65–66, 70–71, 76,
    88, 90, 163, 184
Sevelamer, for
    hyperphosphatemia, 182
Severe primary
    hyperparathyroidism,
    11–17
SHP. *See* Secondary
    hyperparathyroidism
    (SHP)
Sigma 1 subunit, 107
Single-photon emission
    computed tomography
    (SPECT), 58, 71, 76,
    80–81, 98, 100
    Tc-99 m sestamibi SPECT-CT,
        88, 90
Sporadic hyperparathyroidism, 77,
    106, 107, 121, 132–133
Sub-PTX. *See* Subtotal
    parathyroidectomy
    (sub-PTX)
Subtotal parathyroidectomy
    (sub-PTX), 97
    for MEN-1 patients, 77–78
Subtrochanteric femur
    fracture, 11–13
    management of, 14
Superior parathyroid glands, 68
Surgery
    for asymptomatic PHPT,
        4, 5, 7
    for children, 123–124
    for ectopic parathyroid
        glands, 70